Palgrave Studies in Science, Knowledge and Policy

The increasing production of knowledge for governance has resulted in major shifts in governance practices and public policy, especially for the work of knowledge producers and those identified as relevant 'experts'. Given the centrality of knowledge to the governing of contemporary societies, how can we theorise the politics of knowledge for policy and governance and the strategies of policy influence?

Palgrave Studies in Knowledge, Policy and Governance invites social scientists to explore the construction of knowledge and expertise in governance processes across policy fields (e.g. crime, education, genomics, health, migration, sustainability, etc). We support interdisciplinary scholarship that deals with theorising real world issues, as well as practice-based perspectives. Contributors commonly work within Politics, Social Policy and Sociology but we welcome proposals from a wide range of disciplinary settings as well as those working in the policy world. The series encompasses diverse topics, methods and disciplines and we are keen to receive proposals for solo-authored, co-authored and edited books in either standard Palgrave or (shorter) Palgrave Pivot formats.

Please contact the series editors, Sotiria Grek (Sotiria.Grek@ed.ac.uk) and Kat Smith (Katherine.smith.100@strath.ac.uk) to discuss your initial ideas and outline proposals.

Kat Smith is Professor of Public Health Policy at the University of Strathclyde. Dr Sotiria Grek is Senior Lecturer at the University of Edinburgh. They are both members of SKAPE (the Centre for Science, Knowledge and Policy at Edinburgh).

More information about this series at
https://link.springer.com/bookseries/14592

Charlotte Godziewski

The Politics of Health Promotion

In the European Union

palgrave
macmillan

Charlotte Godziewski
Department of International Politics
at City
University of London
London, UK

Palgrave Studies in Science, Knowledge and Policy
ISBN 978-3-030-97869-3 ISBN 978-3-030-97870-9 (eBook)
https://doi.org/10.1007/978-3-030-97870-9

This Palgrave Macmillan imprint is published by the registered company Springer Nature Switzerland AG
The registered company address is: Gewerbestrasse 11, 6330 Cham, Switzerland

For Gabriel

Acknowledgements

This book is the outcome of a six-year research and writing process. I would not have been able to complete it without all the support, mentorship, and help that I received along the way. First, I would like to express my sincere gratitude to the series editors Kat Smith and Sotiria Grek, who generously advised and supported me. A huge thank you to Paul Cairney for taking the time to review and provide helpful feedback on the manuscript, and to the two anonymous reviewers who provided valuable advice on the book proposal. Throughout the research and writing process, I had the privilege to receive guidance from and be inspired by the work of so many thinkers I admire. They include Simon Rushton, Owen Parker, Kat Smith, Ian Bache, Meri Koivusalo, Ellie Brooks, Mary Guy, Ted Schrecker, Tammy Hervey, Louise Dalingwater, Anastasia Shesterinina, Rob Ralston, Lauren Carters-White, Garrett W. Brown and many more. Thank you also to my former colleagues in the Department of Sociology and Policy at Aston University for giving me the space to complete my thesis and work on this book.

I would also like to thank all the interviewees who took part in this research project. Thank you for accepting to put aside an hour, sometimes even more, to kindly share your expertise and insights with me. Thank you to the publishers John Wiley & Sons and Taylor & Francis, for allowing me to draw on material previously published in the following two articles: 'Godziewski, C. (2020). Evidence and Power in EU Governance of Health Promotion: Discursive Obstacles to a "Health in All Policies" Approach. *Journal of Common Market Studies*, **58**(5), 1307–1324'. And 'Godziewski, C. (2021). Is 'Health in All Policies' everybody's responsibility? Discourses of multistakeholderism and the lifestyle drift phenomenon. *Critical Policy Studies*, **15**(2), 229–246'.

Finally, I want to thank my family and friends for their support. A very special thank goes to Gabriel Siles-Brügge. Thank you for your patience and your emotional and academic support.

Contents

About the Author

Charlotte Godziewski is a Lecturer (Assistant Professor) in International Politics at City, University of London. Her research explores the politics of health, with a current empirical focus on the EU. Her doctoral thesis was awarded the 2021 Best Ph.D. Thesis Prize by the University Association for Contemporary European Studies (UACES). Charlotte is a coordinator of 'EUHealthGov', the UACES-funded research network on EU Health Governance.

Abbreviations

AMR	Anti-Microbial Resistance
AVMSD	Audio-Visual Media Services Directive
CAP	Common Agricultural Policy
CDA	Critical Discourse Analysis
CF	Cohesion Fund
CHAFEA	Consumer, Health, Agriculture and Food Executive Agency
CJEU	Court of Justice of the European Union
CSR	Country-Specific Recommendation
DG	Directorate General
DG ECFIN	DG for Economic and Financial Affairs
DG GROW	DG for Internal Market, Industry, Entrepreneurship and SMEs
DG SANTE	DG for Health and Food Safety
DI	Discursive Institutionalism
DNA	Deoxyribonucleic Acid
EC	European Commission
ECDC	European Centre for Disease Control
ECHI	European Core Health Indicators
EFTA	European Free Trade Association
EIB	European Investment Bank
EMA	European Medicines Agency
EMU	European Monetary Union
EP	European Parliament
ERDF	European Regional Development Fund
ESF	European Social Fund
ESIF	European Structural and Investment Fund
EU	European Union

FDI	Foreign Direct Investment
GDP	Gross Domestic Product
HERA	European Health Emergency Preparedness and Response Authority
HIA	Health Impact Assessment
HiAP	Health in All Policies
HLG	High Level Group on Nutrition and Physical Activity
HP	Health Programme
IA	Impact Assessment
IMF	International Monetary Fund
ISG	Interservice Group
JRC	Joint Research Centre
LMIC	Low- and Middle Income Country
MEP	Member of the European Parliament
MFF	Multiannual Financial Framework
NCD	Non-Communicable Disease
NGO	Non-Governmental Organisation
NMG	New Modes of Governance
OECD	Organisation for Economic Co-operation and Development
OMC	Open Method of Coordination
REFIT	Regulatory Fitness and Performance Programme
RRF	Recovery and Resilience Facility
SDH	Social Determinants of Health
SGP	Stability and Growth Pact
SGPP	Steering Group on Health Promotion, Disease Prevention and Management of Non-Communicable Diseases
SMART	Specific, Measurable, Achievable, Relevant, Time-bound
SME	Small and Medium-sized Enterprises
SPS	Sanitary and Phytosanitary
TEC	Treaty of the European Community
TEU	Treaty of the European Union
TFEU	Treaty on the Functioning of the European Union
TTIP	Transatlantic Trade and Investment Partnership
UK	United Kingdom
UNESDA	Union of EU Soft Drinks Associations
WHO	World Health Organisation

List of Figures

List of Tables

List of Boxes

CHAPTER 1

Introduction

How should EU governance contribute to public health, and what role can it realistically play? What is the appropriate scope of EU engagement in public health policy? While the current global COVID-19 crisis has raised health on the political agenda (EU Health Governance Research Network, 2021; European Health Union, 2020), these questions predate the pandemic. The Treaty on the Functioning of the European Union (TFEU) states that the EU has a role in health protection and promotion, yet the implications of the rather vaguely phrased Article 168 TFEU vary widely. In this book, I explore how different ways to think about health affect the perceived scope of 'health promotion'. What is commonly understood as health promotion, then, is not an a priori category, but is constructed (and challenged) politically. To analyse the politics of health promotion at EU level, I focus on the fate of a health mainstreaming agenda introduced in 2006 called 'Health in All Policies' (HiAP). The analysis in this book explores the malleability of the 'HiAP' concept, showing how institutional structures, but also power dynamics related to ingrained ideas and discourses, shape the way(s) in which HiAP becomes (re)defined. As we will see throughout the chapters, these power dynamics reflect tensions around social versus economic EU integration, as well as epistemological tensions in the field of public health.

C. Godziewski, *The Politics of Health Promotion*, Palgrave Studies in Science, Knowledge and Policy, https://doi.org/10.1007/978-3-030-97870-9_1

What role should the EU play in promoting health? What role *can* it realistically play? To approach these questions, we first need to think about the meaning and scope of health promotion. What do we commonly think about when we hear the term 'health promotion', and what can we gain from broadening its definition? What determines how broad is too broad, and when do policies affecting *indirect* determinants of health cease to be considered as relevant to health? This book explores the politics of health promotion at EU level. By 'politics of health promotion', I mean power dynamics which construct the meaning of health promotion, which determines what qualifies as health promotion, which delimits its scope. I focus on the EU because this unique set of institutions offers particularly interesting insights into institutional and ideational tensions between social and economic priorities, between what is considered 'political' and what is considered 'apolitical', and between social and biomedical understandings of health. Despite having limited official health competencies, many of the EU's activities nevertheless impact public health in direct and indirect ways. In that sense, the EU case study sheds light on the extent to which policies *indirectly* affecting health can (or fail to) be perceived as relevant to health.

In 2006, the Finnish EU presidency introduced the concept of 'Health in All Policies' (HiAP) as an attempt to increase awareness and consideration for public health impacts of non-health policy areas. This stems from a now widely researched understanding that societal inequities are harmful to public health, and that much of what shapes public health lies outside of the public health policy domain (the concept of 'macrosocial determinants of health' as I will develop below). In turn, HiAP can be seen as trying to make *a health case* for improving how EU governance affects socioeconomic and environmental inequities—ultimately, a health case for a more social EU.

This book analyses the politics of health promotion at EU level through the lens of HiAP. It shows how HiAP advocates sought to broaden the understanding of what constitutes health promotion, while avoiding (for pragmatic reasons) to explicitly engage with the inherently normative dimension of this endeavour. However, at the beginning of the book, I suggest that we cannot talk about macrosocial determinants of health without talking about the elephant in the room: neoliberalism and its resilience. Yes, decades of invoking 'neoliberalism' has meant it risks becoming a catchphrase of little use (Bell & Green, 2016), and indeed, I seek to challenge the idea that the EU is *monolithically* neoliberal.

However, if macrosocial factors that widen inequalities are considered harmful to health, then it is useful to engage with the dominant rationality that underpins those factors when exploring the nuanced and multifaceted processes through which it operates. The book then explores the ways in which EU institutional asymmetries reproduce a neoliberal logic and render a HiAP uptake (as imagined by Finnish HiAP advocates) difficult. Put simply, the governance areas dealt with in a more binding, hard way pertain to macrosocial determinants of health and have generally the least *perceived* relevance to health. On the other hand, what is commonly perceived as being relevant to health tends to be governed in a much softer, less binding way. Introducing HiAP has proven unable to change this asymmetry.

I argue that, beyond institutional factors, ideational power dynamics explain some of this inability: the ways in which health, health promotion, even NCDs, but also knowledge and evidence are thought about do not lead to a social justice-oriented understanding of HiAP. This goes to the heart of epistemological tensions in public health between biomedical versus social conceptualisations of health. Related to the difficult relationship between public health and politics, and between research and policy, I argue that HiAP is intentionally malleable and vague about its normative roots. While this will have likely helped the concept reaching the EU governance space, it has also resulted in HiAP becoming easily reinterpreted to fit existing structures, rather than challenging and changing them.

Overall, this book aims to demonstrate that the governance of health promotion is political, in the sense that it relates to power dynamics that structure social relations and our understanding of the world (including our understanding of what constitutes health promotion). HiAP tries to challenge those power dynamics and shift the understanding of health promotion towards a more holistic, social justice and sustainability-oriented vision. But it fails to bring about meaningful change within the EU institutional and ideational structures, insofar as it avoids engaging explicitly with the normative, political changes its implementation would require.

1.1 Health and the European Union: Renewed Attention?

The COVID-19 pandemic has raised public health higher onto political agendas, including at EU level. COVID-19 represents an immediate health threat, but the unfolding of the pandemic, and its response, has also highlighted the flaws, weaknesses and fundamental injustices in many political systems (Chang, 2020; Godziewski, 2020; Jones & Hameiri, 2021). For those interested in the workings of the EU, the pandemic provides many useful lessons and insights (Brooks et al., 2020). From sudden travel restrictions even within the Schengen area to the challenges of setting up a joint procurement for vaccines, and the launch of the NextGenerationEU recovery instrument, the past two years have seen some extraordinary measures set up to respond to this extraordinary crisis. Even the fiscal coordination mechanisms were suspended through the triggering of the so-called general escape clause. Pre-pandemic, the fate of the stand-alone EU Health Programme was uncertain to say the least. Now, the new version of a Health Programme—EU4Health—has seen its budget grow from around 449 million (for the 2014–2020 period) to around 5.3 billion euros over the 2021–2027 period (European Commission, 2021). It is fair to say that this book is coming out amid an extremely eventful and changing public health and political context likely to deeply transform the EU's involvement in public health. So, rather than speculating on the future developments and future impacts of recent changes, this book focuses on the time preceding COVID-19 and the extent to which EU institutions have been suited (or not) to considering how their activities impact health indirectly.

Questions around the EU's role in health governance open broader discussions that predate and go beyond the current pandemic response. They invite us to dig deeper than the coronavirus context, and instead apply a *health lens* to the debates of social versus economic EU integration, and to critical EU studies. A holistic understanding of health pushes the boundaries of what can and should be considered a determinant of health. This begs the question: what does 'health promotion' encompass? We know that the causes and effects of the pandemic are influenced by pre-existing societal inequities, and they interact with non-communicable diseases, such as chronic respiratory diseases, cardiovascular diseases and their risk factors like obesity or smoking (Bambra et al., 2020). It is therefore useful to look beyond COVID-19 and ask to what extent the

EU has been shaping these broader determinants of health, whether it has fostered an environment conducive to good health at the population level. A growing body of research shows that public health is affected by political decisions taken in areas that have apparently nothing to do with health: housing policies, welfare systems, urban policies, labour market policies, fiscal governance, trade policies, the agricultural and food system, even broader and more fundamentally than that: the overarching, macroeconomic system and its propensity to widen or reduce societal inequities (Meier et al., 2019).

If these are the factors that (indirectly) shape the health status of populations, considering them seriously has implications for what should count as health promotion. One implication is that the EU has much more influence on public health than is often considered. The old assumption that, given it is a member states competence, public health promotion has little to do with the EU is now increasingly being challenged (Lamping, 2005; Schimmelfennig & Rittberger, 2006). As such, many indirect, macrosocial determinants of health are EU competencies (see European Union, 2016). This justifies the need for more attention to the public health impact of EU (non-health) activities, that is, the need for more HiAP-like thinking at EU level. As will be explained in the following chapter, HiAP is a broad policy agenda which calls for the mainstreaming of health in other policy areas. It is driven by a concern for macrosocial determinants of health and is intended to draw attention to the indirect impact of non-health policies on public health. HiAP was introduced to the EU in 2006 during the Finnish EU presidency, in an attempt to re-emphasise the importance and potential scope of Article 168 TFEU.

1.2 Aim and Argument of This Book

The aim of this book is to explore what happens to an idea like HiAP when introduced at EU level: what are the various kinds of challenges to institutional change towards more consideration of macrosocial determinants of health? The EU is a particularly interesting institutional setting in which to look at this question, precisely because on the one hand its role in health is perceived as limited, yet its influence on indirect, macrosocial determinants of health is considerable, for example through fiscal coordination as well as Single Market integration. This book will explore some of the asymmetrical power dynamics, institutional and ideational, that challenge any institutional change on macrosocial determinants of health. At the same time, the concept of 'HiAP' has been introduced at EU level, despite the limited perceived relevance of the EU to health. How come

HiAP 'made it' to the EU in the first place is another question this book seeks to answer.

Throughout the chapters, we will explore HiAP in the EU institutional, ideational and discursive context. Institutional and ideational context, here, refers to two (co-constitutive) types of structures which shape what is doable and thinkable. Analysing the obstacles to HiAP within the EU *institutional context* refers to analysing how the EU institutional architecture, through its propensity to favour market integration over social protection, affects public health indirectly and affects what HiAP can achieve. Yet institutional structures do not exist out of the blue, detached from social construction. Instead, they are sustained through structuring ideas and systems of meanings. Analysing the *ideational context*—how certain frames and paradigms dominant in the EU and pertaining to how health and knowledge are made sense of—allows us to better understand the cognitive processes that delimit what HiAP can mean and achieve within these institutional boundaries. Finally, the *discursive context* here refers to the agential space in which EU actors can actively define and redefine HiAP, either in ways that fit the dominant structures, or in ways that seek to promote endogenous institutional change. Rather than looking at an exhaustive overview of individual policies and the extent to which they consider health, the focus in this book is on how ideological (in a broad, constructivist sense) power dynamics play out in relation to HiAP in the EU context. The purpose is thus to move away from a technical approach to health mainstreaming, and to embrace the normative essence of HiAP, taking a broad conceptualisation of 'health promotion' as a starting point and analysing how HiAP plays out in the EU.

The central argument developed is that a radical HiAP shift is unlikely to happen in the EU setting, because HiAP is normatively at odds with the dominant neoliberal rationality prevailing at EU level. This is most visible in the asymmetrical EU institutional architecture that systematically privileges market goals over social goals: those EU governance areas that affect macrosocial determinants of health tend to be those areas with the most constraining forms of governance. However, they also have the least perceived relevance to health. In contrast, the areas with the most perceived relevance to health promotion pertain largely to behavioural determinants of health and tend to be governed in a softer, less binding way. However, enabling HiAP is not solely a matter of redressing this constitutional asymmetry. In other words, changing the EU institutional architecture in a way that no longer systematically privileges markets over people does not guarantee that a HiAP shift would easily follow. Instead, it is necessary to also consider the ideational and meaning-making context that prevails at the EU. This is where it becomes interesting to look at paradigms of health and knowledge shape the framing of NCDs and evidence respectively, and how this system of meanings has an impact on the possibility to take up HiAP. For example, we can dig into how the framing of NCDs as a problem mostly related to ageing populations is embedded in an economic paradigm of health and explore the neoliberal underpinnings of this frame. While ideational and institutional structures are of course co-constitutive and reinforce each other, the point here is that the former is more than merely path-dependent consequences of the latter and should be considered in its own right. Yet finally, the fact that HiAP as a concept reached the EU space in the first place suggests that space for contestation and gradual change exists, even if it points to incremental, evolutionary change processes rather than revolutionary, radical ones. Here, I argue that this relative success is due to HiAP being a so-called chameleonic idea (Smith, 2013): it made it into the EU space because its normativity is strategically toned down, and there remains an intentional level of vagueness. The consequence, however, is that the meaning and definition of HiAP is an important site of discursive power struggle, with attempts to co-opt it, make it fit the existing structures and promote institutional continuity, and attempts to recycle HiAP and represent a new version of this old idea to have another try at fostering institutional change. Ultimately, the resilience of neoliberalism goes beyond EU institutional power dynamics and has also to do with ideational paradigms that provide the frames to make sense of the world, as well as active discursive ability. At the same time, these structures are not pre-determined and forever fixed—they can be strategically challenged, and they do evolve, however incrementally.

1.3 Research Approach and Methods

This book is based on research undertaken between October 2016 and January 2020. The empirical analysis is based on document analysis, and insights from 32 semi-structured elite interviews (with a total of 35 participants), undertaken in two rounds. During the first round of interview in Brussels and Luxembourg in 2018 (March–July), I conducted 28 interviews with 29 participants: eight officials of EU health advocacy groups, seven officials of the European Commission (EC) Directorate General for Health and Food Safety (DG SANTE) (six current and one former official), one official of the EC Joint Research Centre (JRC), three officials of the European Parliament (EP) (one member of the European Parliament (MEP), one MEP assistant and one former MEP assistant), five representatives of health ministries of EU member states, four associations representing the interests of the food and retail industry, and one representative of a research and evaluation company.

To follow up on the insights gained in the first round, I conducted a second round of interviews in Finland (Helsinki & Tampere, in April 2019), during which I spoke to seven participants in four interviews. I chose Finland because, besides having a long history with HiAP, Finland is the member state which has introduced HiAP at EU level most prominently during its EU Presidency in 2006. The aim of these interviews was twofold: to better understand the process of introducing HiAP at EU level, as well as the HiAP idea in Finland, nowadays and back when this kind of idea first emerged. The interviewees were three former Finnish health ministry officials who worked on the 'Health for All' agenda in the 1970s and 1980s; two current Finnish health ministry officials (one of whom was already interviewed once in the first round of interviews), one public health researcher and one Finnish health advocate from a non-governmental organisation (NGO).

My approach to interviews was to dialogically bring about understandings of meanings and discourses (Kvale, 1996, pp. 38–46). Rather than a search for factual information only, the interviews allowed me to better make sense of concepts, how they matter, and what their effects are—in a way that would not have been possible to decipher from texts alone. As such, interviews allowed me to seek triangulation, in the sense of combining document analysis and interview data to better understand the relevance of some ideas and some concepts as opposed to others, to interpret 'what matters' (Fielding and Fielding, 1986, cited in Flick, 2018). The interviews and their interpretation guided the development of this research project through 'grounded conceptualisation' (Belfrage & Hauf, 2017). This refers to a double hermeneutic cycle whereby a discursively constructed reality is interpreted by interviewees, and then again by the researcher herself (Furlong & Marsh, 2010, p. 185). That means the research process departed from an initial provisional conceptualisation of an issue (broadly the EU's role in NCD governance) and was modified and re-theorised as a result of fieldwork (with a clearer focus on HiAP).

The semi-structured nature of the interviews provided flexibility to develop broader topics, including the evolution of DG SANTE, the EC's involvement in public health promotion, the role of the EP and latest policy developments in the area. This created a picture in which 'sensitising concepts' (Faircloth, 2012, p. 272) appeared as more important than the original focus, caught my attention and guided the evolution of the research. These concepts were investigated in increasing depth (in two cases, interviewees were contacted a second time to elaborate on the new foci): first, the challenges to implementing HiAP and 'the politics of defining HiAP' in relation to health promotion and NCD prevention. Second, the role of evidence and knowledge in public health promotion: how to process and review it, and how to devise effective assessment methods and identify best practices. Interviewees were split between a majority who firmly adhered to the principle of evidence-based health policymaking, and a few public health policymakers and advocates who highlighted the shortcomings of evidence-based policymaking. Brought to the forefront was the ontological dilemma in public health between aspiring to produce 'normatively neutral' knowledge and recognising that the political and social dimensions of public health elude objectivity. This dilemma appeared to be salient in the attempts to implement HiAP, because HiAP refers to both a normative vision and a technical process. The EU context illustrates these tensions particularly well because of both its 'technocratic' nature and its market-promoting institutional structure.

As mentioned above, the analysis in this book is based on both interviews and documents. Around 280 EU grey literature files were downloaded from the website of the EC, the EP and the EUR-Lex repository, out of which a total of 106 documents (including websites) were subsequently included in the analysis. Given the breadth of the research topic, I collected documents on a variety of topics, which I categorised in the following way (with overlap): DG SANTE Health Programmes and Strategies; chronic diseases/NCDs; HiAP; social determinants of health and health inequalities; alcohol policy; the Audio-visual Media Services Directive (AVMSD); Better Regulation and EC working methods; the Common Agricultural Policy (CAP); the European Core Health Indicators (ECHI); the European Structural and Investment Fund (ESIF); EU Health Policy Forum; the European Semester; the 2006 Finnish presidency; Horizon 2020; EU health knowledge cycles; nutrition and physical activity; occupational health; the Steering Group for health promotion, disease prevention and management of non-communicable diseases (SGPP); EU Social Pillar; tobacco policy; JRC publications; and the 2019 Finnish EU presidency documents. The selection and inclusion of documents were done following a logic of purposeful and emergent sampling (Emmel, 2014). Purposeful, as the selection of texts was done using pragmatic judgement about what is most relevant. Emergent, as the inclusion and selection of documents resulted from the input of interviewees during fieldwork.

I approached the documents and interview texts with a focus on discourse, to identify 'regularities in meanings' (Taylor, 2001, p. 9), and understand how dominant discourse(s) are shaped, reproduced but also contradicted, and how they structure meanings. Concretely, this translated into particular attention to how health and NCDs are talked about and defined; how/in relation to what are they contextualised? Another focus of the discourse analysis was around the meaning of knowledge and evidence: what does the way EU documents talk about evidence say about the assumptions underlying what constitutes reasonable knowledge, and what does that mean for health promotion and HiAP? What counts as useful and useable knowledge? How are certain kinds of evidence legitimised through discourse and in the texts? While discourses are underpinned by normative struggles, they are not merely a vehicle that reflects existing power dynamics. Instead, they need to be understood as producing these normative struggles, reinforcing established norms but also potentially challenging it.

Bacchi (2005) explains that there is a structure/agency tension at the heart of the theoretical conceptualisation of discourse analysis, which relates to 'whether we ought to think of subjects primarily as discourse users or as constituted in discourse' (Bacchi, 2005, p. 200 [emphasis in original]). This tension is seen in the difference between, on the one hand, the critical discourse analysis (CDA) tradition, which tends to be inspired by (neo-)Marxism and neo-Gramscianism and is more concerned with exposing how hegemonic power operates in discourses (see Fairclough, 2003, 2015; Wodak, 2001). This type of analysis is more concerned with the use of rhetoric and linguistic techniques to intentionally maintain power dynamics in a way that benefits the elite (Jorgensen & Phillips, 2002). Implicitly, this approach puts more emphasis on discursive agency to maintain oppressive structures in place. On the other hand, those who tend to consider subjects as 'constituted in discourse' represent the more Foucault-inspired, post-structuralist tradition of discourse analysis. Here, the emphasis is less on the agency of subjects, and more on how discourses produce subjects and produce reality. However even in this approach to discourse analysis, there is still space for agency, insofar as people can be aware of discourses while enacting them or contesting them. While it is important to bear this distinction in mind, I would argue that it should not be taken as a clear dichotomy, and instead, it is useful to negotiate both elements of discursive agency and structure. In the fourth chapter, I talk about how discursive institutionalism can be used to navigate these tensions. It is not possible to know the extent of intentionality versus structure that is taking place in discursive process, but it might be reasonable to assume a degree of overlap between institutional context, ideational structures and discursive agency. As Bacchi (2005, p. 208) concludes:

> In clarifying the distinction between these two analytical projects the goal is not to suggest that they should be kept separate, but that understanding them as two analytical perspectives is a first step to considering how they can be combined.

To understand what discourse analysis consists of here, it is useful to briefly consider the relationship between episteme, statements and discourses (Mills, 1997, pp. 48–76). An episteme represents what is considered at a particular time as counting as knowledge. This is not about what discourse/ideology dominates at a particular time, but rather, much more broadly, what kind of 'knowledge era' we are situated in. A statement can be understood as an 'act of communication' (which can include utterances, behaviours, visuals, symbols, texts, practices…) in its particular meaning context (the same utterance can represent different statements when occurring in different contexts). Sets of statements constitute discourses, and a multiplicity of discourses makes up the contemporary episteme. The purpose of discourse analysis is to make sense of the relationship between statements, discourses and episteme, in a way that seeks to reveal the normative underpinnings of the various elements, how these relate to each other, as well as their contingent nature. The aim of the discourse analysis here in this book is then to explore these relationships in multiple ways: how are framings of things (like 'NCDs' or 'evidence') embedded within broader paradigms which provide the background cognitive landscape for making sense of those things in relation to others? How can discourse be mobilised to shape malleable meaning of ideas? How does appeal to normative neutrality grant authority and legitimacy to certain ideas around health, and not others? These are some of the guiding questions this book explores in relation to the HiAP agenda in the EU.

1.4 Chapter Outline

This book is structured in the following way: in Chapter 2, I start by presenting HiAP; first of all, that requires familiarisation with the 'complexity turn' in public health promotion and NCD research, i.e. the increasing body of research that looks at the social, macroeconomic and political determinants of health—which I refer to as 'macrosocial determinants of health' (Putnam and Galea, 2008, p. 275). This chapter also engages with the notion of neoliberalism as a macrosocial determinant of ill-health, and why it is still relevant to study this, while being aware of the risks of 'neoliberalism' becoming a catch-all term. I then present the HiAP idea within this complexity turn: as an attempt to translate the awareness of macrosocial determinants of health into a policy agenda. HiAP is by no means the only such attempt to bridge research and policy; however, it is the concept that was adopted in the EU, which is the focus in this book. Nor is HiAP only about health promotion and NCD prevention. However, for the purpose of narrowing down an already vast study subject, I focus on considering health promotion and action on the macrosocial determinants of NCDs.

To understand HiAP, Chapter 2 also presents the roots of the concept, which date back to around the time of the Alma-Ata declaration and the WHO Health for All agenda (WHO, 1978, 1981) (at least this is a remarkably important moment in the history of HiAP; however, the idea itself predates even the 1970s). To provide context to the introduction of HiAP at EU level, this chapter also first briefly introduces HiAP in Finland. Indeed, it was the 2006 Finnish presidency that most emblematically raised HiAP onto the EU agenda and looking at their own national journey with HiAP is useful context to understand the EU case study. The final part of this chapter engages with the challenges of researching HiAP, and the shortcomings of an approach focused disproportionately on technical implementation. I conclude the first chapter by arguing for the need to study HiAP from a critical social scientific perspective, and what is more, from a critical political science perspective.

Chapter 3 introduces the EU institutional context and situates the contribution of this book within the EU health literature. Some scholars have theorised the EU's involvement in health by using the notion of 'constitutional asymmetry'. This chapter outlines and engages with the idea that the EU institutions, by virtue of how they developed over time, now present an ingrained bias in favour of economic integration as opposed to social integration, making the EU inherently more of a market-creating endeavour, than a market-correcting one. In turn, a common argument is that the increasing involvement of the EU in health is symptomatic of market rationality spilling over into social areas. This book takes this argument a step further by looking at the obstacles to acting upon macrosocial determinants of health. In an institutional context that seems so ill-fitted to address macrosocial determinants of health (and in which even health policies are arguably not driven by health concerns), how come HiAP became endorsed by the European Council, yet how does it fail to bring about meaningful change? I suggest that the obstacles to a healthier EU include but go beyond constitutional asymmetry and also encompass ideational and discursive power imbalances. The final section of Chapter 3 then offers a map of the EU governance types (soft, hard and meta-regulatory), which will be useful to keep in mind in subsequent chapters.

Chapter 4 explores the tensions around theorising institutional change and continuity, and how to make sense of them in relation to HiAP in the EU. To do so, it briefly introduces discursive institutionalism (DI) as developed by Schmidt (2008, 2015), and how it will be adapted and applied analytically to the study of HiAP in the EU. DI is really an umbrella term for multiple frameworks—the basic tenets being a focus on ideational power to explain institutional change and continuity. It regards institutions as fluid, as both constraining actors and the product of them, and identifies three elements that need to be analysed in order to make sense of endogenous institutional change: institutional context, background ideas and 'foreground discursive abilities'. This book takes a 'structure-heavy' interpretation of DI to group institutional context and background ideas as structures that tend to maintain institutional continuity, and discursive abilities as the space for agency which can push in a variety of directions, with a varying degree of success. Understanding the interplay between these elements of structure and agency sheds light onto why HiAP managed to be introduced at EU level, but also why it failed to bring about meaningful change.

The fifth chapter, and first empirical chapter, is concerned with analysing the space for HiAP within the EU institutional context and considering constitutional asymmetry (Scharpf, 2006). To approach this vast task in a concise and overarching way, I draw on the categorisation of soft, hard and meta-regulatory governance. For each of those categories, I provide examples in relation to which I reflect upon the space for HiAP. Ultimately what this chapter shows is that the EU institutional context is not favourable to HiAP. This, in and of itself, is neither novel, nor surprising. However, the broad conceptualisation of health promotion which considers neoliberalism a determinant of health provides a new picture of how the constitutional asymmetry operates in a way that undermines a normatively meaningful HiAP: what emerges is a picture in which softer governance areas have more perceived relevance to health, but also remain limited to behavioural, individualised (so-called 'proximal') determinants of health, while harder (and meta-regulatory) governance areas—which are actually the areas that impact 'distal', macrosocial determinants of health—remain perceived as irrelevant to health.

Although constitutional asymmetry is clearly an important way in which neoliberal rationality is reproduced and which undermines a normatively meaningful HiAP, leaving the analysis there would fail to capture numerous other dynamics, and whole other parts of the story. This leads to Chapter 6, which explores the ideational landscape, the 'background ideational structures' that shape HiAP. The point here is that these ideational reproductions of neoliberalism need to be considered as more than merely the consequence of institutional configuration. Chapter 6 thus delves into analyses of paradigms and frames (Ruston & Williams, 2012) around health as well as around knowledge and evidence. It teases out how this web of ideational structure limits the way health promotion can be understood and how HiAP can be imagined. By looking at the impact of a predominantly economic paradigm of health on the framing of NCDs, and of a narrow definition of what constitutes legitimate evidence on the normativity and complexity of a concept like HiAP, this chapter suggests that the asymmetrical dynamics at EU level favouring neoliberal rationality are not only a matter of institutional architecture, but also of ideational architecture.

Despite this less than propitious structural environment, HiAP still managed to become 'a thing', a concept referred to at least in some parts of the EC. This in and of itself suggests that, while EU institutions tend to reproduce a neoliberal market rationality, they do not do so monolithically, and, visibly, some space for contestation exists. Yet

HiAP simultaneously succeeded in reaching the EU space and failed to bring about meaningful change. This space for agency—however flawed or limited—is the focus of Chapter 7. Instead of thinking of institutional and ideational structures as completely rigid, pre-determined and only ever changing as a result of exogenous shocks, foreground discursive abilities are the spaces in which agents from within the institutions can articulate discourses that are critical (or not) of their own institution. This does not mean that radical change is around the corner. Instead, what Chapter 7 reveals is that HiAP is a so-called chameleonic idea (Smith, 2013). This means it is intentionally malleable and normatively vague, to become more easily accepted in those spaces it would normally challenge. However, chameleonic ideas are by definition easy to co-opt, water down or redefine. In this chapter, I explore the various forms and evolutions that HiAP takes at EU level, and which all together illustrate the political struggle to define HiAP—from watered-down forms that seek institutional continuity (e.g. multistakeholder HiAP) to recycled versions of HiAP represented by the next Finnish EU presidency (in this case: the economy of wellbeing theme of the 2019 EU presidency). The final section reflects on the potential of the co-existence, along chameleonic ideas like HiAP, of more radical ideas which I argue nevertheless share a common normative basis, like degrowth.

References

Bacchi, C. (2005). Discourse, discourse everywhere: Subject "agency" in feminist discourse methodology. *Nordic Journal of Women's Studies, 13*(3), 198–209.

Bambra, C., Riordan, R., Ford, J., & Matthews, F. (2020). The COVID-19 pandemic and health inequalities. *Journal of Epidemiology and Community Health, 74*(11), 964–968.

Belfrage, C., & Hauf, F. (2017). The gentle art of retroduction: Critical realism, cultural political economy and critical grounded theory. *Organization Studies., 38*(2), 251–271.

Bell, K., & Green, J. (2016). On the perils of invoking neoliberalism in public health critique. *Critical Public Health, 26*(3), 239–243.

Brooks, E., De Ruijter, A., & Greer, S. (2020). Covid-19 and European Union health policy: From crisis to collective action. In B. Vanhercke, S. Spasova, & B. Fronteddu (Eds.), *Social policy in the European Union: State of play 2020. Facing the pandemic* (pp. 33–52). Brussels, European Trade Union Institute (ETUI) and European Social Observatory (OSE).

Chang, D. (2020, April 17). Coronavirus: Normal was the problem. *Ecologist*. https://theecologist.org/2020/apr/17/coronavirus-normal-was-problem. Accessed 17 September 2021.

EU Health Governance Research Network. (2021). Welcome to the EU Health Governance Network. *Webpage*. https://euhealthgov.org. Accessed 17 September 2021.

European Commission. (2021). Regulation (EU) 2021/522 of the European parliament and of the council of 24 March 2021 establishing a Programme for the Union's action in the field of health ('EU4Health Programme') for the period 2021–2027, and repealing Regulation (EU) No 282/2014. https://eur-lex.europa.eu/legal-content/EN/TXT/PDF/?uri=CELEX:32021R0522&from=EN . Accessed 04 May 2022.

European Health Union. (2020). Manifesto for a European Health Union. *Webpage*. https://europeanhealthunion.eu. Accessed 17 September 2021.

European Union. (2016). *Division of competences within the European Union. Summaries of EU Legislation*. https://eur-lex.europa.eu/legal-content/EN/TXT/?uri=LEGISSUM%3Aai0020. Accessed 12 November 2019.

Emmel, N. (2014). Purposeful sampling. In N. Emmel (Ed.), *Sampling and choosing cases in qualitative research: A realist approach* (pp. 33–44). Sage.

Fairclough, N. (2003). *Analysing discourse: Textual analysis for social research*. Routledge.

Fairclough, N. (2015). *Language and power* (3rd ed.). Routledge.

Faircloth, C. A. (2012). After the interview: What is left at the end. In J. F. Gubrium, J. A. Holstein, & A. B. Marvasti et al. (Eds.), *The SAGE handbook of interview research: The complexity of the craft* (2nd ed., pp. 269–278). Sage.

Flick, U. (2018). Triangulation. In N. K. Denzin & Y. S. Lincoln (Eds.), *The SAGE handbook of qualitative research* (5th ed., pp. 777–804). Sage.

Furlong, P., & Marsh, D. (2010). A skin not a sweater: Ontology and epistemology in political science. In D. Marsh & G. Stoker (Eds.), *Theory and methods in political science* (3rd ed., pp. 184–210). Palgrave Macmillan.

Godziewski, C. (2020, May 27). *As long as economic growth remains the EU's main objective, it will not be well prepared for health threats*. LSE EUROPP Blog. https://blogs.lse.ac.uk/europpblog/2020/05/27/as-long-as-economic-growth-remains-the-eus-main-objective-it-will-not-be-well-prepared-for-health-threats/. Accessed 17 September 2021.

Jones, L., & Hameiri, S. (2021). COVID-19 and the failure of the neoliberal regulatory state. *Review of International Political Economy*. https://doi.org/10.1080/09692290.2021.1892798

Jorgensen, M., & Phillips, L. (2002). *Discourse analysis as theory and method*. Sage.

Kvale, S. (1996). *InterViews*. Sage.

Lamping, W. (2005). European integration and health policy: A peculiar relationship. In M. Steffen (Ed.), *Health Governance in Europe: Issues, Challenges and Theories* (pp. 18–48). Routledge.

Meier, P., Purshouse, R., Bain, M., Bambra, C., Bentall, R., et al. (2019). The SIPHER consortium: Introducing the new UK hub for systems science in public health and health economic research. *Wellcome Open Research, 4*(174). https://doi.org/10.12688/wellcomeopenres.15534.1

Mills, S. (1997). *Discourse*. Routledge.

Putnam, S., & Galea, S. (2008). Epidemiology and the macrosocial determinants of health. *Journal of Public Health Policy, 29*, 275–289.

Rushton, S., & Williams, O. D. (2012). Frames, paradigms and power: Global health policy-making under neoliberalism. *Global Society, 26*(2), 147–167.

Scharpf, F. (2006). The joint-decision trap revisited. *Journal of Common Market Studies, 44*(4), 845–864.

Schimmelfennig, F., & Rittberger, B. (2006). Theories of European integration. In J. Richardson (Ed.), *European Union: Power and policy-making* (3rd ed., pp. 71–93). Routledge.

Schmidt, V., (2008). Discursive institutionalism: The explanatory power of ideas and discourse. *The Annual Review of Political Science, 11*, 303–326.

Schmidt, V. (2015). Discursive institutionalism: Understanding policy in context. In F. Fischer, D. Torgerson, & A. Durnova (Eds.), *Handbook of critical policy studies* (pp. 171–189). Edward Elgar.

Smith, K. E. (2013). *Beyond evidence-based policy in public health: The interplay of ideas*. Palgrave Macmillan.

Taylor, S. (2001). Locating and conducting discourse analytic research. In M. Wetherell, S. Taylor, & S. J. Yates (Eds.), *Discourse as data: A guide for analysis* (pp. 5–48). Sage.

WHO. (1978). *Declaration of Alma Ata*. International Conference of Primary Health Care. https://www.who.int/publications/almaata_declaration_en.pdf. Accessed 11 September 2019.

WHO. (1981). *Global Strategy for health for all by the year 2000*. https://iris.wpro.who.int/bitstream/handle/10665.1/6967/WPR_RC032_GlobalStrategy_1981_en.pdf. Accessed 11 September 2019.

Wodak, R. (2001). What CDA is about—A summary of its history, important concepts and its developments. In R. Wodak & M. Meyer (Eds.), *Methods of critical discourse analysis* (pp. 1–13). Sage.

CHAPTER 2

What Is 'Health in All Policies'?

To understand HiAP, it is necessary to discuss how public health research, especially around non-communicable diseases (NCDs), has been increasingly focused on social, macroeconomic and political determinants of health—so-called macrosocial determinants of health (Putnam & Galea, 2008). Examples include research on trade liberalisation (Koivusalo et al., 2021), corporate political activities (Mialon, 2020; Knai et al., 2018) and austerity measures (Schrecker & Bambra, 2015), all of which have been linked to worsened public health outcomes. What these insights reveal is that determinants of health are far more complex and more political, than the common focus on individual behaviour would suggest. HiAP represents an attempt to bridge research and policy, to translate the awareness to macrosocial determinants of health, into a policy agenda. It is by no means the first attempt to do so, and it is useful to look at the roots of the concept and historically contextualise its introduction at EU level. Understanding the idea's normative roots illuminates epistemological tensions which will be explored throughout the coming chapters. I conclude this chapter by arguing that HiAP is an evidence-informed *political* endeavour, and that we therefore need to study it from a (critical) social scientific perspective.

C. Godziewski, *The Politics of Health Promotion*, Palgrave Studies in Science, Knowledge and Policy, https://doi.org/10.1007/978-3-030-97870-9_2

2.1 The Complexity Turn in Non-Communicable Diseases and Health Promotion

NCDs are responsible for the largest burden of deaths, diseases and disability worldwide (Sheldon & Wright, 2020), including in the European Region. They are sometimes also referred to as 'chronic diseases' and include cardiovascular diseases, diabetes, cancer and chronic respiratory diseases (though some also include mental illnesses in the classification). According to the WHO (2018a), NCDs are responsible for 41 million deaths each year (71% of all deaths globally), 15 million of which qualify as 'premature deaths' (occurring between the ages of 30 and 69). The largest proportion of premature deaths from NCDs occur in low- and middle-income countries (LMIC) (WHO, 2018a). Nevertheless, in the EU in 2016, an estimated 790,000 people died prematurely due to smoking, alcohol consumption, unhealthy diets and/or physical inactivity (European Commission, 2017a). NCDs also increase the risk of developing more severe symptoms of COVID-19 (The Lancet, 2020). It is fair to say that NCDs are one of the most important contemporary public health issues. They are also particularly interesting to study from a critical social scientific perspective, because individual cases are determined by what has often been argued to be modifiable risk factors. This means that, while some risk factors cannot be modified (such as age, sex and other genetic predispositions), to a large extent, NCDs are supposed to be preventable and determined by 'lifestyle' dimensions, such as smoking, diet, and physical activity. This is precisely why HiAP is particularly and strikingly relevant in the context of NCDs. Even though public health messages promoting 'healthy lifestyles' have been around for decades, NCDs are still on the rise, and it is widely understood that tackling them will require political commitment, rather than merely health education campaigns and incentives to change individual behaviours. These political commitments need to be taken overarchingly, and reflected in all policy areas, hence the need for HiAP. Since the start of the pandemic, NCDs, COVID-19 and socioeconomic inequalities have been conceptualised as a 'syndemic' reinforcing health inequalities (Bambra et al., 2020; The Lancet, 2020). The public health community often calls for the generation of more evidence to understand how these public health issues operate and what works best in terms of policy response to NCDs (Horton, 2013; Sacco et al., 2013). While these are still relevant agenda, arguably now the language is shifting more towards justice, political commitment and accountability, which reflects the acknowledgement that simply knowing and conveying what policy approaches would work best does not guarantee its uptake (Zuccala & Horton, 2020).

To understand some fundamental conceptual division lines in public health research, it is useful to examine Labonté's (1998) three levels of health paradigms. He argues that there are broadly three different ways of thinking about health in relation to the 'proximity' or 'distance' to the individual. The first one is the biomedical paradigm, which sees health from the perspective of the body and its pathophysiology. The second one is the behavioural paradigm, which makes sense of health as determined by risks stemming from the way people behave. Finally, the third paradigm is the social one, which thinks of health as determined much more broadly, i.e. as related to the social conditions of life (Labonté, 1998). To give a simple example, diarrhoea seen from a biomedical perspective will be concerned with the toxicological mechanisms induced by a pathogen in the body. The behavioural lens might focus on hand hygiene to prevent diarrhoea. The social paradigm will look at the social roots of lack of access to water and sanitation infrastructures, such as poverty and social exclusion as a 'social determinant of diarrhoea'. This idea of health paradigms, and close versus remote aetiology, is perhaps most well known in the context of the Dahlgren-Whitehead rainbow model (Dahlgren & Whitehead, 2021). This model layers determinants of health according to their spatial distance from the body, with the closest determinants of health comprising of biological factors (age, genetics, etc.), followed by behavioural determinants, social determinants and then, overarchingly, environmental, cultural, political and macroeconomic conditions. Those factors that are perceived as somehow far removed from the individual (i.e. macroeconomic, social and political factors) have been termed distal or 'macrosocial' determinants of health (Huynen et al., 2005).

The 'complexity turn' in NCD and health promotion is characterised by more engagement with the kinds of determinants of health that have been deemed farther away removed from individuals (social and macrosocial). The rainbow model has been influential in paving the way towards more consideration for macrosocial (or 'distal') determinants of health. However, the distal/proximal and upstream/downstream metaphor, despite having gained a lot of traction, does not necessarily evoke the same things to everyone (McMahon, 2021). Furthermore, Krieger (2008) warns against the danger of the proximal/distal (also referred to as 'upstream/downstream') categorisation to conflate time, space, level and strength of causality. Indeed, though these 'distal' determinants of health might be spatially removed from the body, they can still affect health in very direct and tangible ways (she uses the example of abortion legislation). It is also important to consider the political economy relating the different 'levels' and avoid wrongly conceptualising a linear relationship in which distal determinants of health only matters indirectly by affecting the 'real' proximal determinants down the line. In this book, reference to 'macrosocial' determinant of health will be favoured over 'distal determinants of health', to avoid those conflations. To be very clear, when I refer to macrosocial determinants of health, I mean the policies, governance systems and power dynamics that shape inequities, including via the distribution of income and wealth. While something like housing conditions and education level can be classified as a social determinant of health, the macrosocial determinants of health as referred here relate to the characteristics of political systems that affect inequities in society (which then result in housing inequalities, among other social conditions)—i.e. the political causes of housing inequalities, rather than the housing inequalities themselves. And when I talk about health promotion policies targeted at proximal determinants of health, I mean primarily behavioural health promotion, such as education campaigns, information (including food labelling) and 'nudging' policies (Baum & Fisher, 2014).

Public health budgets tend to be driven disproportionately by a biomedical conceptualisation of health, which relates more to 'proximal' explanations of ill-health and focuses on curing disease, i.e. a focus on healthcare, rather than preventing disease through public health promotion (Stuckler et al., 2010). This reflects concerns of financial sustainability of *healthcare* systems, but also presents more obviously lucrative opportunities, mostly for the pharmaceutical and medical device industry, compared to socially driven health promotion (Schrecker & Bambra, 2015). In the field of NCDs, the biomedical paradigm of health takes the shape of, for example, innovative agenda for personalised medicine and health technologies. The biomedical response to the NCD burden has been criticised mostly for failing to address, and sometimes even for worsening, inequities in health (Frankford, 1994; Glasgow & Schrecker, 2016). Indeed, as will be developed in more depth below, the NCD burden has much to do with health inequities and their determinants. Biomedical responses to NCDs can exacerbate those inequities by targeting high quality, highly personalised treatments preferentially at those who can afford them.

Alongside the accent on treating and curing diseases, disease prevention and health promotion have been most thought about in relation to individual behaviour. A behavioural approach to health promotion typically includes providing information, health education on the one hand (teaching individual people how to adopt a healthy lifestyle) as well as nudging policies on the other hand. Nudging policies are small incentives put in place to subconsciously nudge the individual towards a healthy lifestyle. For example, nudging policies for healthy diet promotion can include putting fruit and vegetables at the entrance of the supermarket while 'hiding' junk foods at the back. The idea is to send subliminal messages to invite the consumer to choose the healthy option (Alemanno & Garde, 2015). A disproportionately strong focus on behavioural approaches has been criticised for putting the blame on individuals while ignoring, even obscuring, structural factors that cause the NCD burden by, among other things, leading to these behaviours. The suggestion that health inequalities are the result of poor behaviour is misleading and stigmatising (Glaze & Richardson, 2017; McCartney et al., 2013). It is now a widely held position in the public health field that behavioural, nudging interventions are not only inefficient, but can often be actively harmful, especially as it tends to be used as a substitute for action on macrosocial determinants of health. Van Den Broucke (2014) argues that behavioural paradigms have been misused and that, when combined with action on the social determinants of health and when used properly (including, for example, on politicians and policymakers themselves), they may still have a lot to offer. The most important issue with behavioural nudges and education campaigns is their use to actively deter from other (macrosocial) public health measures, the unfair blaming that results from this instrumental and short-sighted view of health promotion.

The Social (and Political) Determinants of Health

In summary, both biomedical and behavioural paradigms of health have been strongly criticised on the grounds that the NCD 'crisis' is a political, socioeconomic one, and that biomedical and behavioural solutions represent merely a superficial plaster on a much bigger problem, which actively deters policymakers from looking at the root causes of the population's illnesses (Glasgow, 2005; Ottersen et al., 2014). The notion that public health is socially and politically determined has a long history. In Europe, the observation that health is determined by social and living conditions emerged at least as early as the nineteenth century, with public health scientists like Rudolph Virchow in Germany (Mackenbach, 2009) and Louis-René Villermé in France (Lynch, 2020, p. 48). This understanding informed the post-World War II development of more comprehensive welfare states in Western European democracies. The Black Report was published in the UK in 1980 by the Department for Health and Social Security, in an attempt to explain the structural causes of health inequalities (Townsend et al., 1992). The report showed that working-class men were twice as likely—and women two and a half times more likely—to self-report long-standing illnesses (Townsend et al., 1992, p. 198) compared to wealthier groups. It also stressed that, even though infant mortality had decreased in each social class between the 1960s and 1970s, the inequality in infant mortality between social classes had grown during that period (p.198). As a possible explanation, the authors of the report stated that '*in our view much of the evidence on social inequalities in health can be adequately understood in terms of specific features of the socio-economic environment* [*emphasis in original text*]' (p. 199). Acknowledging specific areas worth improving, like ante-natal care, they claimed that 'there is undoubtedly much that cannot be understood in terms of the impact of so specific factors [like ante-natal care], but only in terms of more diffuse consequences of the class structure: poverty, working conditions, and deprivation in its various forms' (p. 199).

Unfortunately, and unsurprisingly, the recommendations of the report were not given much weight under Thatcher's premiership. However, the awareness and understanding of the link between poor health and poverty, as well as the link between poor health and inequalities, were there. A second report, the 'Health Divide', was published with updated information about health inequalities in the UK (Townsend et al., 1992). A growing amount of research sought to document the state of health inequalities and the impact of social inequalities on health (Kickbusch, 2003; Marmot, 2005; Whitehead, 1991). This debate led to the adoption of the term 'social determinants of health' (SDH), which refers to social inequalities (related, for example, to employment and housing conditions) at the root of health inequalities (Marmot, 2015). It explains why people with lower socioeconomic status tend to have worse health conditions than wealthier people with better living and working conditions, and that these differences are visible along a 'social gradient', rather than them being attributable simply to a link between poverty and disease. In 2005, the WHO launched a Commission on Social Determinants of Health, led by Sir Michael Marmot (WHO, 2008). In line with the notion that inequalities in SDH lead to unfair and avoidable health inequalities, i.e. health inequities (as opposed to individual genetic variations), and that health is a human right and a goal in itself, those researching SDH are calling for more health equity (Lawn et al., 2008; Marmot, 2018). The terms inequity and inequality are generally used in the literature in the same way as Evan et al. (2001): 'Inequalities in health describe the differences in health between groups independent of any assessment of their fairness. Inequities refer to a subset of inequalities that are deemed unfair' (Evans T. et al., 2001, p. 4). The COVID-19 pandemic has also revived the call for more action on health inequalities, with research highlighting the syndemic effects between gendered and capitalism-induced inequities, NCDs and COVID-19 (Bambra et al., 2020).

While more vulnerable and poorer groups have worse health outcomes compared to wealthier population groups, inequity itself may indeed be harmful for the whole of society, not merely for the poor (Wilkinson & Pickett, 2010, 2018). Wilkinson and Pickett (2010, 2018) argue that inequity in societies leads to worse mental health throughout all social classes, for example via increased 'class anxiety' (the pressure to display an image of belonging to a high social class). This class anxiety encourages the consumption of so-called positional goods, an unfulfilling consumption which can leave people anxious and may even decrease the sense of meaning in life (Büchs & Koch, 2019; Jackson, 2018). Furthermore, unequal societies have more markedly differential dominance behaviour system responses, whereby a stark gap between 'dominant individuals' and 'submissive individuals' is associated with narcissism and maniac behaviour for the former, and anxiety and depression for the latter (Wilkinson & Pickett, 2018). While Wilkinson and Pickett's key argument has faced criticism on methodological grounds, the point to consider here is that the negative health effects of inequalities should not be conflated with the negative effects of poverty on health (Smith, 2013a).

The Turn to Complexity

The social—and I would add *political*—paradigm of health is the kind of paradigm that allows thinking about and potentially addressing the kinds of root causes of contemporary public health issues. Evans and Stoddart explain the concept of SDH with a thermostat analogy (Evans & Stoddart, 1990 cited in Schrecker & Bambra, 2015, p. 7). They explain how one way to react to chilly temperatures inside a house is to turn up the thermostat and spend more on heating. Similarly, governments that focus too narrowly on the medical paradigm of health will respond to population's health issues by increasing the healthcare budget, up to a point where they consider it unaffordable. Instead, Evans and Stoddart point out that to keep the house warm, one can also invest in well-insulated walls and double-glazed windows, after which there is no need to increase the heating as much anymore. Instead of wondering 'how can we build more high-tech radiators?' (biomedical paradigm) or 'how do we teach people to knit warm blankets?' (behavioural paradigm), we need to focus on 'what prevents investing in double glazing, who/what is responsible for the cold in the first place, and how can this change?' (social and political paradigm). Applied to the case of health, this would mean looking at the possibilities for investing in health promotion and mental, physical, social, environmental and spiritual wellbeing more broadly, by improving the living and working conditions of the population and understanding the challenges to do so. Ultimately, this relates to wealth and income redistribution, through public spending and regulation, not least of capital. This kind of agenda promotes health equity and considers socioeconomic conditions as the root determinants of health, but also emphasises the link between environmental sustainability and health equity (Evans et al., 2001).

This kind of agenda also leads to a 'complex' understanding of health promotion, as it zooms in on the multiple, interrelated, indirect root causes of poor public health. 'Complexity' here refers first and foremost to the recognition that health is shaped to a large extent indirectly, and that various aspects of the world and society, such as various kinds of inequity, the environment and globalisation, intersect. The section above introduced some of the research that looks at the relationship between social inequities and health. Research in the field of political science of health, or the sociology of health, has looked at the complex interlinkages between public health and other societal dimensions: globalisation, international political economy and health (Koivusalo, 2014; Labonté et al., 2011), patriarchy and health (Daykin & Naidoo, 1995; Hammarström & Ripper, 1999; Rogers, 2006), racism, post-colonial theory and health (Douglas, 1995; Paradies, 2016), intersectionality theory and health (Hankivsky &

Christoffersen, 2008; Lapalme et al., 2019), or the relationship between environmental and human health (Watts et al., 2018; Zinsstag et al., 2011). Thinking about health promotion merely in terms of individual behaviour incentives, then, reflects a lack of understanding of complexity. If public health is shaped by so many complex and interacting political, economic and social factors, then health promotion should be about much more than incentivising healthy individual behaviour. This is, in essence, what characterises the 'complexity turn' in NCDs and health promotion. A complex understanding of health promotion recognises the intersection between environmental, animal and human health, and the relationship between these facets of planetary health and oppressive political systems. The complexity turn also goes hand in hand with a recognition of normativity and political nature of health promotion and NCD prevention. Indeed, if contemporary public health issues are very complex, then solving them through a purely technical approach will not be possible. Instead, one needs to recognise and embrace the fact that public health is political.

2.2 Translation into Policy: The HiAP Agenda in the EU

Along with explaining the macrosocial determinants of health, researchers have developed recommendations on how this knowledge could be applied to policymaking. One approach that is being advocated for by an increasing number of public health researchers and experts is 'Health in All Policies' (HiAP). It is the approach that has been put forward at EU level under the Finnish presidency in 2006 and which is still referred to now in the EC. The following section will explain what HiAP is, the story of how it emerged in Finland and how researchers have studied it so far. It concludes by explaining how it was put on the EU agenda in 2006.

Broad, so-called intersectoral public health promotion approaches have regained attention. Such approaches are not new, but they are becoming more and more mainstream and increasingly accepted including within the policymaking sphere. And, as we will explore, they have changed along the process. Concepts like 'healthy public policies', 'intersectoral action for health', 'whole-of-government approach' and HiAP are all efforts to move beyond narrow individual behaviour framings of health promotion. While there are variations between these approaches, broadly one of their main common messages is the call for a holistic, integrative vision that takes into account the health impact of other policy areas and a call for a mainstreaming and prioritising of health and wellbeing promotion as a goal in and of itself, one that other sectors need to work towards. Some researchers have looked at how to shift the discourse from health inequality/inequity, which they term a 'pathogenic' approach, towards a discourse of health equality/equity—a 'salutogenic' approach (Mittelmark et al., 2017). They argue that the former focuses on risk, ill-health and disease, and that such a rationale is problematic because it tends to see good health as the normal, default state of being and ill-health an abnormal state in need of fixing. This results in a minimalist approach to public health and a neglect of health promotion, given that it starts from the assumption that unless actively harmed, the default is that people are healthy. In a pathogenic paradigm, health promotion fails to clearly differentiate itself from disease prevention, and health promotion really is reduced to disease prevention done at an earlier stage (Antonovsky, 1996). In salutogenesis, on the other hand, sees health/illness as a continuum rather than a binary, and prioritises the creation of population health and wellbeing, seeking ways for policies to maximise health (Rouvinen-Wilenius et al., 2019). It recognises that a laissez-faire stance in public health governance and in relation to macrosocial determinants of health does not safeguard good health, because of the propensity of that stance to exacerbate societal inequities. As such, the normative ideal of HiAP echoes a salutogenic understanding of population health and wellbeing, rather than a pathogenic one.

HiAP has been defined as:

> an approach to public policies across sectors that systematically takes into account the health and health systems implications of decisions, seeks synergies and avoids harmful health impacts, in order to improve population health and health equity. A HiAP approach is founded on health-related rights and obligations. It emphasizes the consequences of public policies on health determinants and aims to improve the accountability of policy-makers for health impacts at all levels of policy-making. (Leppo et al., 2013, p. 6)

It is driven by a view of health as a human right and a matter of social justice. It implies that the economy should work towards attaining high levels of wellbeing, health and environmental sustainability, rather than the other way around. In 2013, HiAP was the theme of the eighth global conference on health promotion. The conference resulted in the Helsinki Statement on Health in All Policies, as well as a HiAP Framework for country action (WHO, 2013, 2014a). In that context, HiAP is a term that has been taken up by the WHO, which since then published recommendations and guidelines for implementation (WHO, 2015a, 2018b). While examples drawing on this general idea could already be found in various countries, the conference gave HiAP a global significance and proposed a common concept and a common language for this conversation (Tang et al., 2014). HiAP is now drawn upon in many different countries, including Finland, Canada, Ecuador, Thailand and Australia (Ståhl et al., 2006; WHO, 2014a). In Ecuador, for example, social policies are required to take into consideration the 'Plan Nacional para el buen vivir', which saw social investment increase 2.5 times between 2006 and 2011 (WHO, 2014a, p. i21). Since the 2013 Helsinki Statement on Health in All Policies, the WHO is providing support for HiAP implementation, such as how to identify (or create) structures and processes for HiAP, and how to build human resource capacity (WHO, 2014a, 2015b, 2018b; for concrete examples and technical guidance for HiAP implementation, see also WHO, 2014b). These three components: structures, processes and capacity, were also the ones most emphasised by one of the interviewees involved in the HiAP plan of the 2006 Finnish EU presidency.

The Story of HiAP in Finland

HiAP is arguably the most prominent example of 'broad health promotion approaches' prevalent in the EU currently. HiAP is relevant to virtually every health-related topic, and it is therefore not possible to comprehensively study it in all its aspects at once. Yet NCDs prevention and health promotion, because of their relevance to broad and political, macrosocial determinants, are a good focus to analyse the normative aspects of HiAP. To get a better understanding of the roots and development of the HiAP idea, it is useful to look at the story of HiAP in Finland. This story is informed in large part by in-depth semi-structured interviews[1] undertaken in Helsinki and Tampere in April 2019. It explains the historical context in which this way of thinking about health and its relevance to other policy areas emerged. It also includes a section about the structures and processes for HiAP in Finland and how they, too, have been evolving over time.

In the first half of the twentieth century, Finland was considered one of the European countries with the worst health status. After World War II, a significant proportion of school children were undernourished. UNICEF got involved in programmes to provide essential fatty acids and other sources of nutrients to improve the Finnish children's health status. Nowadays, the country's social and health model, along with the ones of similar Nordic countries and their so-called Nordic, social democratic welfare model (Esping-Andersen, 1990), is often regarded as being among the most progressive and efficient in the world. Finland underwent profound structural transformations that have led to dramatic improvements in its population health and wellbeing. The concept of 'Health for All by 2000', which was developed at WHO level and in which Finland was particularly active, was a key catalyst of this transformation. Health for All, most Finnish interviewees agreed, was the precursor of HiAP. In fact, HiAP is seen as 'an attempt to translate this health policy [approach, i.e. Health for All] into EU language'.[2]

To understand HiAP, it is therefore helpful to look at the precursor of the concept: 'Health for All (by 2000)' (WHO, 1981). The idea of 'Health for All by 2000' started in the WHO in the 1970s. It reflects a normative vision for health that emphasises the social nature of health, considers health as a human right and recognises that all public policy areas have an impact on determinants of health (Mahler, 1981). The global strategy for Health for All was launched by the adoption of the famous Alma-Ata declaration (WHO, 1978, 1981). This concept resonated very strongly in Finland, which managed to raise it high on the national agenda at that time thanks to the mobilisation of both medical doctors and politicians. The development of Health for All by 2000 took place simultaneously at national level and at WHO level, notably under the three-term (1967–1982) regional directorship

[1] Interviews with two former high-level officials in the Finnish ministry of health, one former Finnish member of Parliament, two current officials from the ministry of health and social affairs, and one health advocate in a Finnish NGO.

[2] Quoted from interviewee 31.

for WHO Europe of Finnish public health scholar Leo Kaprio (Johns Hopkins Bloomberg School of Public Health, n.d.). Finland was seen as one of the pioneer countries in committing to the WHO's Health for All Programme (Melkas, 1988).

At the national level, the success of this idea was, in addition to the merits of the concept in and of itself and the science behind it, dependent on the traction gained within the social democratic party at the time. Health for All came in the context of a general move towards socially progressive, left-wing governance and the 'radical' ideas that characterised the 1960s more generally across many Western countries. The Health for All idea was reflected in a series of progressive welfare reforms that took place in the 1970s and 1980s (Finnish Ministry of Social Affairs and Health, n.d.). The approach to implementing it was to break it down into separate topics (nutrition, road traffic, tobacco, etc.) and then act upon them comprehensively, on multiple fronts. Melkas (2013) and Leppo (1988) provide a systematic historical account of the journey of HiAP in Finland since that time (Leppo & Melkas, 1988; Melkas, 2013). There was a 'rural to urban' dynamic whereby the projects started to be put in place in the rural and deprived areas of the country and were then gradually spread out to reach cities as well. One flagship initiative was the North Karelia Project in 1972. It took a broad community-based approach to improving cardiovascular health in a small community (Jousilahti, 2014). The interviewees explained that while in win–win situations, 'low-hanging fruits' were useful and important to seize, confrontation and resistance against conflicting interests were also indispensable. They highlighted the necessity of taking a strong normative stance on policy issues relevant to health, even when the stance was deemed very unpopular at first. That was the case, for example, in the road safety context. Between 1973 and 1978, several health policy measures were taken to improve road safety and reduce the number of deaths and injuries due to road traffic accidents. Speed limits were lowered, compulsory helmets for motorbikes were introduced, as well as compulsory seat belts in cars. These measures faced vehement opposition by several important lobby groups, including the car industry. Simultaneously, road infrastructures were improved, including the construction of broad cycling and pedestrian lanes. Opposition against these public health measures had to be confronted, and mindsets had to change. However, by the time clear and significant health benefits started to be visible, the general attitude towards these measures among the population improved. The interviewees explained that to bring about meaningful changes like these, patience is needed, but also strong and trustworthy institutions. The police, for example, were an ally in getting the road safety agenda through. The political system in Finland which tends to result in broad coalitions was also mentioned as one factor which facilitated the continuity and long-term vision for Health for All, as well as a long-standing culture of lively civil society activism.

On the international scene, Finland was actively involved in the Health for All agenda at the WHO Regional Office for Europe. While Finland was not alone in this endeavour, the link between Finland and the WHO European region was key in raising the concept of Health for All both nationally and internationally, and to amplifying Finland's voice in the global health arena. Health targets were developed in the WHO in the framework of the Health for All project, which allowed countries to gain more accurate information on the health status of their population, which at that time was very new. What was crucial was that the international Health for All agenda was also thought to serve an additional purpose: to promote peace. One interviewee in particular explained that, with health representing a terrain of relatively low political and diplomatic sensitivity, the Health for All agenda was indeed also used to try to improve diplomatic relations. The rationale was that peace is a basic pre-requisite for a healthy population, and that is how the concept was expanded as an avenue for dialogue in the Cold War context. This East–West diplomatic stance was important for Finland, a small Nordic country with long border with the then Soviet Union. In later parts of the book, one important dimension that will be explored is the normativity HiAP, and the problems with arguing for health instrumentally, to promote economic growth for example. Interestingly, health is drawn upon instrumentally here, too, albeit for a different end.

What came out very clearly from the interviews undertaken with those people who were involved in the Finnish Health for All agenda, and what needs to be emphasised here, is the normative essence and political driver of Health for All. These public health measures implemented were driven by scientific evidence, but the political support was also key. In the international context, the core human rights and social justice values also played a major role. Arguably, it seems like the economic paradigm of health as a means to promote growth, and health as a 'cost-effective investment', may not have dominated at that time and in that particular context, or at least not to the same extent. This is very important to point out because it already shows fundamental differences between how HiAP 'got started' in Finland pre-1990s and how HiAP got started in the EU.

With respect to HiAP and fostering intersectoral collaboration for health promotion, Finland and the Nordic countries, more generally, have often been seen as forerunners. The previous section has already shed some light on the historical context which led Finland to develop structures and processes that facilitate—to some extent—a HiAP way of working. Ståhl and Lahtinen (2006) explain how the preparation of the Finnish National Health Report took place in 2006, and how the 2006 report differed from previous ones. The Finnish National Health Report is published every four years, towards the end of the national government's cycle. This allows for the evaluation of the government's degree of success in promoting health and wellbeing and serves as an agenda-setting document for the next government. The preparation of the 2006 report considerably strengthened the intersectoral collaboration through the creation of a new process called the 'bilateral dialogue'. Here, all the various ministries meet with the Health and Social Affairs Ministry for an in-depth discussion and evaluation of the relevance of their own policy agenda to the population's health and wellbeing, and the role of health in their decision-making processes (Ståhl & Lahtinen, 2006). The outcomes of the new report preparation process were the establishment of new structures for intersectoral collaboration on health, such as the Advisory Board for Public Health, which included a division specialised in intersectoral cooperation (Ståhl & Lahtinen, 2006).

Another avenue for strengthening intersectoral collaboration across ministries, and including parliaments and government, was indeed in some ways (and perhaps paradoxically so) the 1995 accession to the EU (Kokkinen et al., 2019; Ståhl & Lahtinen, 2006). Important coordination efforts were made to ensure the preparation of coherent national positions with respect to EU matters. Those efforts included setting up new structures: 35 sectorial preparatory subcommittees that bring together various policy areas around one issue. The subcommittees have a restricted, ministerial-only composition and a broader composition in which stakeholders can provide input. Proposals from these subcommittees need to be adopted in the government's and in the parliament's relevant committees (Ståhl & Lahtinen, 2006; Taipale, 2018). It may thus be suggested that Finland has comparatively robust structures that allow intersectoral collaboration and allow health to be brought to all tables. This was also the opinion of one of the Finnish health policymakers interviewed.

> I think that in some respects [related to intersectoral action for health] Finland has been very strong and a forerunner, including in trade and health for example. [...] the openness that used to exist in the ministry to consider health also plays a role. [...] There was an astonishing change, back in 2014 when we were working on the HiAP strategy at national level, the high point for me was the meeting of all secretaries from all secretariats, they all got together for a full day – including the prime minister, the minister of health etc. They sat the whole day to discuss how health should be included. We thought that that was a major success. It was exactly the time when you could have said 'this is how HiAP should be done'[...] (Quote from interviewee 31)

However, that same person also recognised the growing challenges to protect these structures and to ensure they are used to promote public health:

> [...] But actually, it [i.e. the outcome of the meeting mentioned in the quote above] turned out the exact opposite, the main thrust was to have health service and health technology as a major contributor of economic growth, that was the main point from the ministry of health and social affairs. That was a shock, we were so ready for it, we had prepared so much for many years, we got everyone together... (Quote from interviewee 31)

Indeed, more critical research is examining the effects of welfare restructuring that has been taking place in Finland since the early 1990s recession (Kokkinen et al., 2019). It suggests that Finland has not been immune to the global neoliberal trends and has seen its HiAP-like social wellbeing and health model gradually eroded: the institutionalisation of prioritising economic interest (of the top few) over social wellbeing occurred through various administrative reforms, such as one which conferred decision-making regarding budgets related to healthcare and social affairs on the ministry of finance (and away from the ministry of social affairs and health). The culture of lobbyism also started to gain traction, especially since the EU accession in 1995 (Kokkinen et al., 2019). As of 2019, the Advisory Board for Public Health (mentioned in the paragraph above) was no longer active, even though its legal basis still exists (WHO, 2015c).

Another example of the effect of neoliberal reforms in the 1990s in Finland on the potential to implement HiAP is the changing relationship between the central government and municipalities (Virtanen et al.,

2016). The Finnish state has a history of conferring much autonomy to municipalities. They are responsible for delivering most social services, including healthcare and education, as well as land-use planning, and the overall prosperity of the municipality (Nousianen, 2018). They also have a legal requirement to undertake a health impact assessment (HIA) for every new policy project. In addition to the budget provided by the central government, municipalities levy taxes, including corporate and real estate taxes. The central government is responsible for evening out the disparities between municipalities (Nousianen, 2018). This special relation between central government and municipalities has been seen as a strong advantage for implementing HiAP in a way that takes into account local needs, while being guided by the government's overarching strategic vision for HiAP. However, since 1993, state subsidy reforms 'dismantled the state's strong normative steering mechanism over municipalities' (Kokkinen et al., 2019, p. 4). The budget coming from the central government to municipalities was gradually reduced and no longer ear-marked. Municipalities were encouraged to outsource and privatise traditionally public services, including parts of the healthcare services. The absence of strategic steering, budget cuts and the fragmentation of service provision have made the adoption of HiAP in Finland much more difficult.

The 2006 Finnish EU Presidency

Finland joined the EU in 1995. As mentioned in the section above, the 1990s was also a period of economic recession in Finland, which ushered in a range of neoliberal austerity reforms (Kokkinen et al., 2019). In many ways, Finland's EU accession did not facilitate the protection of the country's social interests. Indeed, it has been argued by multiple critical voices that, while EU membership came with many advantages and progress, the policy space for health was reduced as a result of EU membership. This was perhaps most visible in Finnish alcohol policies (Ollila, 2011; Shankardass et al., 2018). Alcohol policies traditionally have had a strong public health dimension in Finland (and other Nordic countries) which was challenged by the strictly Single Market approach taken by the EU. Finland was not the only member state who had to work hard to protect the public health logic of their alcohol policies. The other two EU Nordic member states experienced similar situations (Holder et al., 1998). Ultimately, however, the message from some interviewees was that while EU competencies can sometimes provide additional challenges, it is often still possible (for certain countries at least) to simultaneously protect public services and public health measures and comply with EU laws, provided enough time and capacity are available to member states. For example, the national government retained a selling monopoly on both gambling and alcohol.

In 2006, Finland held the EU Presidency and introduced HiAP as one of its main themes. This decision stemmed from a concern that the EU was not doing enough to respect Article 168 of the TFEU. Indeed, Article 168 suggests that the EU has had an entry point for mainstreaming HiAP since the 1990s, and as such, the Finnish presidency did not introduce something entirely new and unheard of (Merkel, 2010).

> You realise that you have in the Treaty, not only a mandate but a requirement to protect health. And that was seen as a major tool in maintaining health and especially public health, while keeping health systems off the EU agenda. (Quote from interviewee 31)

The EU, thus, has a mandate to implement HiAP. The case for health mainstreaming is stated in Article 168 TFEU and is further strengthened by Article 9 TFEU which, under the heading 'Provisions having general application', states that:

> In defining and implementing its policies and activities, the Union shall take into account requirements linked to the promotion of a high level of employment, the guarantee of adequate social protection, the fight against social exclusion, and a high level of education, training and protection of human health. (Article 9 TFEU)

Furthermore, the establishment of the Health Strategy 'Together for Health', was said to represent an explicit and legitimate commitment from the EC to mainstream health objectives in all its actions (Merkel, 2010). Despite the thin legal basis, growing understanding of the intersectoral nature of health has led to a growing awareness of how the EU nonetheless influences population health, for example through shaping determinants of health (European Commission, 2013a; Goldner Lang, 2017; Jarman & Koivusalo, 2017; Karanikolos et al., 2013; Koivusalo, 2010; Ollila et al., 2006; Ståhl et al., 2006). The idea that health is shaped outside the health policy area and that it is necessary to foster an intersectoral approach to health promotion was well understood and oftentimes stated in interviews with officials from DG SANTE:

> I think when you're looking at the issues like health determinants or disease prevention and health promotion, I think it's important to remember that it is a multi-faceted thing and that it's not one measure that's going to change the situation. [...] You have to look at the entire picture I think and that's where of course changing lifestyles is very difficult because of different factors intervening and different cultural aspects, different economic aspects, and it's only by taking a holistic approach that you can hope to make any progress over time. (Quote from interviewee 28)

However, the extent to which health was taken into consideration across EU actions so far has not been satisfactory and needed (still needs) to be improved. This prompted the Finnish team to adopt this concept for their 2006 presidency. The accent was put on health protection and promotion, and the way it was shaped was intended to be a continuation of Health for All. One of the interviewees explained that the EC was keen to take HiAP further, beyond the Finnish presidency. HiAP was welcomed by the EU Council at the Employment, Social Policy, Health and Consumer Affairs Council meeting, during which all of the core messages of HiAP were stressed: a recognition that health is valuable per se, that it is not merely a matter of personal choice, and that health determinants are shaped largely in policy areas outside the health sector. The Council conclusions invited the EC to set out a plan to implement it and include it in its Health Strategy, as well as to improve the knowledge base and identification of the EU policies that have an impact on health (EU Council, 2006a). The conclusions also reminded early EC commitments from the 1990s to consider health in other policy areas. A second set of Council conclusions reiterating the commitments to HiAP was published in 2010 (EU Council, 2010). The 2017 Companion Report published by DG SANTE, for example, puts forward as its first conclusion the need to address the SDH, the vicious circle between ill-health and poverty and that this action requires multi-sectoral collaboration (European Commission, 2017a). At the time of the Finnish presidency, it was also very clear that HiAP was something that needed to be put in place across EU institutions. Finland had another EU presidency during the second half of 2019, in which the social and health theme was to introduce the concept of 'wellbeing economy'.

2.3 Researching HiAP: A Technical and Political Task

Ideas like HiAP reflect the growing awareness of the social drivers of health, recognising that all public policy areas can have an impact on health directly or indirectly. Rather than disciplining and nudging people's behaviour, HiAP aims for a deeper societal transformation by tackling the social root causes of health inequalities. To illustrate with a few examples, a HiAP implementation in principle could consist of strengthening the welfare system and improving redistributive policies, promoting healthy and safe urban environments, fighting social exclusion and discrimination based on race, gender, sexuality and ability, and working towards a sustainable food system. Rather than a step-by-step guide, HiAP is normatively driven and exhorts a deeper, meaningful political change towards prioritising societal health and wellbeing (Leppo et al., 2013). However, in practice, this kind of more radical transformations is not the kind of changes associated with efforts to implement HiAP. In simple words, how come HiAP fails to bring about radical change, despite its proponents being quite clear about how far-reaching it is supposed to be? How is HiAP both radical and non-radical at the same time? This book wants to focus on the politics, and political economy, of HiAP to explore these issues.

This focus is motivated by the idea that a hypothetico-deductive problem-solving approach will not be able to fully capture how these power dynamics operate. As early as 1991, Kickbusch (1989) argued for the need to develop an 'ecological approach to public health' as an epistemology capable of adequately making sense of the Ottawa Charter of Health Promotion (see WHO, 1986), capable of dealing with complexity, with patterns that 'elude simple models of causality and intervention' (Kickbusch, 1989, p. 265). An ecological understanding of public health would take into consideration the reciprocity between the environment and human health, both of which represent social resources. She argues that an ecological model for health has the potential to bring about dialogue between natural and social sciences. Public health, in those terms, is both the science and the art of promoting health. Generally, there is an awareness, or at the very least a suspicion, that causality and evidence in the way they are conceptualised in positivist natural sciences are ill-equipped to be applied to SDH and political determinants of health. In many cases (though not necessarily, as we've seen before), the more 'distal' the causes analysed, the more difficult it becomes to establish 'causal evidence' links in the way laboratory conditions would allow. It is especially important to engage with the questions of causality when mindful of avoiding the conflation between level, distance and strength of causality (Krieger, 2008). There has been a growing engagement with these epistemological dilemmas within public health and the politics of evidence (Parkhurst, 2017). For example, the point has been made that blind emphasis on evidence can deter from crucial questioning of the purpose and nature of the evidence (Taipale, 2002). Others have argued that a technocratic understanding of evidence can precipitate action towards what is measurable rather than what is desirable, and indeed steer actions more towards behavioural interventions (Smith, 2013a). Even a 'mainstream' established institution like the WHO Commission on SDH recognises that traditional understanding of evidence is not adequate in the case of SDH ('using "evidence" in the narrow causal link sense would be a recipe for doing nothing' [Friel & Marmot, 2011, p. 229]), and takes a broader approach to what constitutes evidence, including indirect links (e.g. if participatory governance is shown to improve housing conditions and improved housing conditions improve health, then it is taken that participatory governance improves health).

HiAP is both a health mainstreaming approach to policymaking and an overarching political project (Leppo et al., 2013; Ståhl et al., 2006). Due to this duality, HiAP carries an inevitable level of vagueness, and its meaning requires contextual adaptation. With the recognition that all policy areas impact on health, HiAP opens up a terminological 'Pandora's box' of what qualifies as public health promotion, and whether 'health' remains an appropriate term when used in such an all-encompassing way (Synnevåg et al., 2018). Admittedly, such use of language runs the risk of being perceived as 'health imperialistic' (Banken, 2001; Kemm, 2001). In response to fears of health imperialism, it is useful to adopt a more fluid understanding of health as physical, mental, social, cultural and spiritual wellbeing as deriving from a commitment to social justice. Later parts of the book will go back and reflect upon the adequacy of staying with the term 'health', and whether talking about 'societal wellbeing' might be more appropriate. These tensions between theoretical conceptualisation as a political, normative project and practical implementation as policy mainstreaming raise questions as to how HiAP should best be studied, and this has implications for how HiAP will be understood and advocated for.

HiAP as Policy Mainstreaming

Many HiAP researchers interested in the policymaking process have used Kingdon's multiple streams model (Baum et al., 2014; Cairney et al., 2021, p. 26; Kingdon, 2014; Leppo et al., 2013; Mauti et al., 2019; Ollila, 2011). This model has been adopted by the WHO, as well as in the context of HiAP in Australia (Kickbusch et al., 2014; WHO, 2015b). Baum et al. (2014) propose a combination of methodological and theoretical tools to evaluate HiAP in South Australia taking into account complexity. Combined with Kingdon's system theory, they use programme logic modelling to measure the health outcomes of the HiAP agenda in South Australia. Their methodology aims to identify HiAP's impact on population health without using statistical inference isolating causal links, acknowledging that this is an inadequate way of researching complex social issues. Rather, they seek to accumulate 'a burden of proof'. What their findings suggested is that health benefits of HiAP were present but fairly limited, which they argue is reflective of the limited budget dedicated to implementing HiAP. They point out that the actions were limited to 'low-hanging fruits' and obvious win–win situations, mostly pertaining to the links between environmental policies, urban planning and health. The SDH, however, the root causes of much of the health burden which are traced back to power, money and resources, were left untouched by HiAP. The authors partly explain this through the fact that local governments do not have the means to meaningfully modify those areas. This points to a problematic situation in which HiAP is mostly attempted to be implemented at a local level. The very idea that HiAP is something for local government only already betrays a narrowing down of the concept and goes against the 'essence' of HiAP.

How an *essence* is supposed to be inculcated into policymaking processes relates to the notion of HiAP as a mainstreaming agenda. Much of the mainstreaming literature focuses on gender mainstreaming, rather than health. Research on gender mainstreaming in the EU was particularly prominent in the early 2000s, when EU new modes of governance (NMGs), the social 'open method of coordination' (OMC) and other meta-policy tools were being developed (Beveridge et al., 2000; Bruno et al., 2006; Jacquot, 2010; Pollack & Hafner-Burton, 2000; Verloo, 2005). Mainstreaming something into policymaking is intended to be about more than only policy content, but also very much about the process (True, 2003). In the case of gender, for example, mainstreaming is not about developing more policies about including women (although this is also likely to be part of the results), but it is about 're-invent[ing] processes' (True, 2003, p. 371) and changing norms. Changing norms is a potentially radically transformative ambition; however, mainstreaming should also be contextualised within the rise of EU NMG, and seen for what it *also* is: a technocratic 'meta-policy instrument' intended to coordinate and rationalise public policy (Halpern et al., 2008). This has not necessarily been successful in achieving its aims: 'unintentional' implications of the EU gender mainstreaming agenda have been to make this policy field 'softer', i.e. less tangibly protected by law (Jacquot, 2010). Similarly to HiAP, then, gender mainstreaming seems to fall prey to a discrepancy between conceptual development and practical implementation (Daly, 2005).

To study HiAP as a normative health mainstreaming project intended to change institutional norms, we need to focus on mainstreaming as a 'meaning-making process' and analyse how it affects established understandings of reality perpetuated by structures and agents. This means looking at the interplay between regularity and idiosyncrasy, between path dependency and contingency, and how meanings are produced and reproduced (Bacchi & Eveline, 2010). Meanings attached to certain concepts, and the practices of creating knowledge, constitute power which shapes, in an ever-evolving way, the essence of concepts (in this case 'HiAP') by shaping what is 'thinkable' and 'sayable'. In other words, HiAP needs to be studied as a process, and this requires a particular approach. As noted by Jacquot (2010) in relation to EU gender mainstreaming: 'In order to trace the effects of mainly soft, informal, and cognitive instruments like gender mainstreaming, analysis cannot be reduced to a focus on traditional, vertical and regulatory change' (Jacquot, 2010, p. 132). As such, these tools develop a kind of life of their own, and it is worth looking at how it differs nowadays in the EU, compared to perhaps more 'vernacular' meanings and usages of HiAP elsewhere and at a different time, and how its meaning is an ever-evolving site of power struggle. A focus on the non-fixed nature of meanings also allows us to explore spaces for contestation and agency, suggesting that the idea's evolution does not happen in a vacuum, but via active discursive practices. At the same time, existing and dominating worldviews and ideational structures also constrain the meanings of HiAP as it enters the EU space.

HiAP as a Political Project

A few HiAP researchers have engaged more explicitly with the politics of HiAP, and they tend to call for a stronger emphasis and more research in that area (Mikkonen, 2018; Oneka et al., 2017). Baum (2007), for example, argues that public health needs to be more engaged with the role of individualistic ideology, the way it suits powerful interests and how it dismisses any collectivist rationale as 'Nanny State'. Koivusalo (2014) explores the policy space for health and HiAP in the light of the politics of international trade and investment agreements. Another example is Labonté's (2014) work on the HiAP relevance of foreign policy. The HARMONICS project looks at barriers to implementing HiAP and includes a stronger focus on politics and power, engaging notably with the consequences of neoliberal reforms on the space for HiAP in Finland mentioned earlier (Kokkinen et al., 2019; Shankardass et al., 2018).

While the HiAP literature has yet to engage more seriously with the political ramification of that idea, there already exists a rich literature on the politics of health, especially on *neoliberalism* and health. This is relevant here because, if we were to follow the HiAP logic all the way through purely as a thought process, the general understanding is that we would end up with policies that radically challenge many of the neoliberal principles, especially in terms of redistribution, regulation and public spending. There are many ways to define neoliberalism: as an ideology, as a set of economic policies or as 'governmentality' (Sadler & Lloyd, 2009). These differing approaches emphasise different dimensions and/or differ in their theoretical underpinnings, but they tend to share a similar logic. Arguably, its strongest principle is 'the conviction that the only legitimate purpose of the state is to safeguard individual, especially commercial, liberty, as well as strong private property rights' (Thorsen & Lie, 2006, p. 14). It regards promoting free markets as both the best and most natural way to organise social life. Practically, this thinking translates into five key tenets: minimal government intervention, market fundamentalism, risk management, individual responsibility and inevitable inequality (Ericson et al., 2000, cited in Ayo, 2012, p. 99). Another fundamental aspect emphasised mostly by those looking at neoliberalism from a governmentality perspective is the intrusion of market rationality into all other spheres of life and the shaping of responsible, entrepreneurial citizens. Consequently, neoliberalism is not so much about mere deregulation, and more about the creation of free markets, with free individuals expected to behave in a way that makes the free market work.

More than just being adopted as a governance rationality, the basic neoliberal premises have gained a status of 'common sense' or 'inevitability' (Peck & Tickell, 2007). At the same time, neoliberalism changes and does not manifest in the same way in different places, which makes it simultaneously an obvious and an elusive, intangible concept. Peck and Tickell (2002) have looked at the transformative and adaptive capacity of neoliberalism and prefer to think of it as a process—neoliberalisation (Peck & Tickell, 2002). The model they came up with to describe some developments of neoliberalism was the two consecutive phases: 'roll-back' neoliberalisation (anti-regulation) and 'roll-out' (meta-regulation) neoliberalisation. The first phase started to take hold following the 'stagflation' crisis in the 1970s and 1980s, the State was rolled back in countries that embraced neoliberalism, and post-World War II welfare institutions were weakened. This was then followed since the 1990s by a 'roll-out' phase along the lines of 'third way neoliberalism'. The new concern was on how to make this governance palatable to the citizens, by presenting it either as an opportunity for responsible citizens or an inevitability (see also Sparke, 2020). Neoliberalisation, Peck and Tickell (2002) argue, is difficult to resist because solutions offered to problems induced as a consequence of the roll-back phase reinforce and are part of the neoliberal project (instead of resisting it). This idea applies to health and neoliberalism, as Sparke (2016) defines contemporary global health formation as:

> the formation of a field of research, intervention and outcomes in which we see micro neoliberal innovations in personalized health risk management frequently being advanced as answers to the destructive legacies of macro neoliberal structural adjustment. (p. 239)

Broadly speaking, the literature on neoliberalism and health tends to fall into one of the three overlapping categories: health in relation to the macro-level of global neoliberal processes, to the meso-level of local (austerity) policies and/or to the micro-level of individual responsibilisation and neoliberal governmentality. In terms of global processes, research has explored how the economic globalisation has affected equity of SDH in the world (Labonté & Schrecker, 2007a, 2007b, 2007c; Lee et al., 2009). Research on the global trade system looks at the impact of free trade agreements on policy space for health (Jarman & Koivusalo, 2017), including via investor protection mechanisms (De Ville & Siles-Brügge, 2017). Others have focused on the growing power of transnational food corporations and the financialisation of the food system, and how this heavily contributed to the nutrition transition and threatened food security (Clapp, 2016; Hawkes, 2005; Hawkes et al., 2009).

Other work has focused more on how these neoliberal processes translate into lived experiences and local policies and impact health. Austerity, beyond its failure to redress the economy in the aftermath of crises, also has devastating effects on health (Kentikelenis et al., 2011; Stuckler & Basu, 2013). More than economic shocks alone, it is the austerity response in combination with economic crises and a lack of social protection that harms population health most severely (Karanikolos et al., 2013; Schrecker & Bambra, 2015; Stuckler et al., 2017). The removal of a safety net and stress induced by economic hardship, precarity of employment and high stress jobs have concrete impacts on health on a public health scale (Schrecker & Bambra, 2015). In contrast, redistributive policies and generous welfare systems have systematically been linked to better health outcomes (Bambra & Eikemo, 2009; Navarro & Shi, 2001; Navarro et al., 2006). Schrecker and Bambra (2015) go so far as to claim that NCDs could be thought of as 'communicable' after all, through the geographical spread of neoliberal ideology. They argue that the harmful health effects of neoliberalism are also transmitted intergenerationally, through the reduction of social mobility, ever-deepening social inequalities and the stereotyping/stigmatisation of some social groups. Echoing a similar rationale, Sell and Williams (2020) talk about a 'structural pathogenesis' to make sense of the relation between political systems and ill-health.

The disproportionate emphasis placed on behavioural health promotion, too, relates to neoliberalism (Allender et al., 2006; Ayo, 2012; Bell K. and Green, 2016; Crawshaw, 2013; Vander Schee, 2007, 2009). Educating and disciplining citizens to behave in a health-conscious way and to aspire to 'healthy lifestyles' illustrate very well what Foucault described as 'governmentality': a technique of governing at a distance that simultaneously promotes individual freedom (by not intervening in citizens' lives too much via regulation) but at the same time disciplines the individuals to 'freely' behave in a way that is deemed responsible (Rose,

N. et al., 2006). This manifestation of neoliberal power at the micro-level not only deters from considering the political causes of ill-health, but it also tends to marginalise and stigmatise certain population groups. The very medicalisation of fat bodies also contributes to making obesity a personal, moral failure (Evans & Colls, 2009; Schorb, 2013).

Working with the term 'neoliberalism' is difficult, because it can be an overstretched, catch-all concept, almost to the point of becoming a cliché (Bell & Green, 2016). Despite this risk, I still think it is worth using this concept, as long as it is done so in a well-defined and nuanced way. A good example is Julia Lynch's latest book on Regimes of Inequality (2020). Lynch (2020) moves beyond 'simply' pointing out where neoliberal rationality impacts on inequality and health. Instead, she provides a sophisticated analysis that considers the interplay of structure, agency and framing, to show how the resilience of inequality is not simply due to neoliberalism, but also to how certain taboos were institutionalised as a result of how centre-left politicians sought to reframe the issue of inequality. The dominant framing of 'health inequality' may well have been an attempt to find a pragmatic, realistic and feasible way into pushing for more social justice, but it ended up having the opposite effect: those framings pushed even further away the possibility of breaking the taboos that redistribution, public spending and market regulation have become (Lynch, 2020). These findings and their parallel with HIAP will be returned to in Chapter 7, when discussing the nature, strategy and 'level of radicality' of HiAP as an idea.

2.4 Conclusion: The Need for a Critical Approach to HiAP

This chapter has introduced some of the basic premises on which the remainder of this book rests: first, that NCDs are an important public health issue, including in the EU; that NCDs are shaped most importantly by factors outside the narrowly defined public health policy field, i.e. factors that shape societal inequity even at a very remote level; and that, based on this understanding, it is important to mainstream health—including health promotion and NCD prevention—into other policy areas. These concerns led to the development of the HiAP policy agenda. Focusing on Finland as an important forerunner of the HiAP approach who brought the concept to the EU, we explored the normative and political roots of the concept, which can be traced back (at least) to the

1970s and the Alma-Ata declaration and the Health for All agenda. We also looked at how Finland managed to set up certain structures and processes to facilitate HiAP, while at the same time challenging those very structures and values in the aftermath of the 1990s recession and the neoliberal reforms that subsist (and perhaps worsen) until today. The last section of the chapter engaged with the debate on how to research HiAP, on the duality between its technical and political aspects, and what it means to be a 'mainstreaming' project. While there is an increasing awareness of the shortcomings of the orthodox public health positivist ontology among HiAP researchers, there is still a lack of engagement between the HiAP scholarship and the critical scholarship on neoliberalism and health.

The link between neoliberal ideology and population ill-health is well documented, and the purpose of the book is not to investigate *if* neoliberalism affects population health. Rather, it takes that relationship as a given, and it takes as a given that the normative HiAP ideal is not compatible with the main tenets of neoliberalism, and instead seeks to explain *how* neoliberalism restricts the space for mainstreaming health in EU governance, and how HiAP proponents deal with this reality. Recognising neoliberalism as a determinant of (ill-)health should lead to a radical reconceptualisation of 'health promotion', making it much broader. This is what this book seeks to explore. In the coming chapters, we will look at manifestation and reproduction of institutional, as well as ideational and discursive barriers to HiAP. Before we go there, the next chapter introduces *the EU context* into which HiAP was introduced. The EU has a mandate to implement HiAP, and HiAP was explicitly put onto the EU agenda. Yet we will see that because of its technocratic and economic growth-driven nature, the EU is a particularly interesting place to critically analyse the political obstacles to HiAP.

References

Alemanno, A., & Garde, A. (Eds.). (2015). *Regulating lifestyle risks: The EU, alcohol, tobacco and unhealthy diets*. Cambridge University Press.

Allender, S., Colquhoun, D., & Kelly, P. (2006). Governing the working population through workplace health: Knowledge, self and power in workplace health programs. *Critical Public Health., 16*(2), 131–142.

Antonovsky, A. (1996). The salutogenic model as a theory to guide health promotion. *Health Promotion International, 11*(1), 11–18.

Ayo, N. (2012). Understanding health promotion in a neoliberal climate and the making of health conscious citizens. *Critical Public Health., 22*(1), 99–105.

Bacchi, C., & Eveline, J. (Eds.). (2010). Mainstreaming and neoliberalism: A contested relationship. In C. Bacchi & J. Eveline (Eds.), *Mainstreaming politics: Gendering practices and feminist theory* (pp. 39–60). University of Adelaide Press.

Bambra, C., & Eikemo, T. A. (2009). Welfare states regimes, unemployment and health: A comparative study of the relationship between unemployment and self-reported health in 23 European countries. *Journal of Epidemiology and Community Health., 63*(2), 92–98.

Bambra, C., Riordan, R., Ford, J., & Matthews, F. (2020). The COVID-19 pandemic and health inequalities. *Journal of Epidemiology and Community Health, 74*(11), 964–968.

Banken, R. (2001). *Strategies for institutionalizing HIA* (ECHP Health Impact Assessment Discussion Paper Number 1).

Baum, F., & Fisher, M. (2014). Why behavioural health promotion endures despite its failure to reduce health inequities. *Sociology of Health and Illness, 36*(2), 213–225.

Baum, F. (2007). Cracking the nut of health equity: Top down and bottom up pressure for action on the social determinants of health. *IUHPE – Promotion & Education, 14*(2), 90–95.

Baum, F., Lawless, A., Delany, T., Macdougall, C., Williams, C., Broderick, D., Wildgoose, D., Harris, E., Mcdermott, D., Kickbusch, I., Popay, J., & Marmot, M. (2014). Evaluation of Health in All Policies: Concept, theory and application. *Health Promotion International, 29*(S1), 130–142.

Bell, K., & Green, J. (2016). On the perils of invoking neoliberalism in public health critique. *Critical Public Health, 26*(3), 239–243.

Beveridge, F., Nott, S., & Stephen, K. (2000). Mainstreaming and the engendering of policymaking: A means to an end? *Journal of European Public Policy, 7*(3), 385–405.

Bruno, I., Jacquot, S., & Mandin, L. (2006). Europeanization through its instrumentation: Benchmarking, mainstreaming and the open method of co-ordination...toolbox or Pandora's box? *Journal of European Public Policy., 13*(4), 519–536.

Büchs, M., & Koch, M. (2019). Challenges for the degrowth transition: The debate about wellbeing. *Futures, 105*, 155–165.

Cairney, P., St Dennis, E., & Mitchell, H. (2021). The future of public health policymaking after COVID-19: A qualitative systematic review of lessons from Health in All Policies. *Open Research Europe*. https://doi.org/10.12688/openreseurope.13178.1

Clapp, J. (2016). *Food* (2nd ed.). Polity Press.

Crawshaw, P. (2013). Public health policy and the behavioural turn: The case of social marketing. *Critical Social Policy, 33*(4), 616–637.
Dahlgren, G., & Whitehead, M. (2021). The Dahlgren-Whitehead model of health determinants: 30 years on and still chasing rainbows. *Public Health, 199*, 20–24.
Daly, M. (2005). Gender mainstreaming in theory and practice. *Social Politics, 12*(3), 433–450.
Daykin, N., & Naidoo, J. (1995). Feminist critiques of health promotion. In R. Bunton, S. Nettleton, & R. Burrows (Eds.), *The sociology of health promotion: Critical analyses of consumption, lifestyle and risk* (pp. 59–69). Routledge.
De Ville, F., & Siles-Brügge, G. (2017). Why TTIP is a game-changer and its critics have a point. *Journal of European Public Policy, 24*(10), 1491–1505.
Douglas, J. (1995). Developing anti-racist health promotion strategies. In R. Bunton, S. Nettleton, & R. Burrows (Eds.), *The sociology of health promotion: Critical analyses of consumption, lifestyle and risk* (pp. 70–77). Routledge.
EU Council. (2006a, 30 November and 1 December). *Council conclusions on Health in All Policies (HiAP)*. 2767th Employment, social policy, health and consumer affairs. https://ec.europa.eu/health/ph_projects/2005/action1/docs/2005_1_18_frep_a8_en.pdf. Accessed 12 November2019.
EU Council. (2010, June 8). *Council conclusions on equity and Health in All Policies: Solidarity in health. 3019th Employment, social policy, health and consumer affairs*. https://www.consilium.europa.eu/uedocs/cms_data/docs/pressdata/en/lsa/114994.pdf. Accessed 12 November 2019.
European Commission. (2013a). *Health inequalities in the EU – Final report of a consortium*. Consortium lead: Sir Michael Marmot. https://ec.europa.eu/health/sites/health/files/social_determinants/docs/healthinequalitiesineu_2013_en.pdf. Accessed 12 November 2019.
European Commission. (2017a). State of Health in the EU: Companion Report 2017. https://ec.europa.eu/health/sites/health/files/state/docs/2017_companion_en.pdf. Accessed 12 November 2019.
Esping, G. (1990). *The three worlds of welfare capitalism*. Polity Press.
Evans, B., & Colls, R. (2009). Measuring fatness, governing bodies: The spatialities of the Body Mass Index (BMI) in anti-obesity politics. *Antipode, 41*(5), 1051–1083.
Evans, T., Whitehead, M., Diderichsen, F., Bhuiya, A., & Wirth, M. (Eds.). (2001). *Challenging inequities in health: From ethics to action*. Oxford University Press.
Finnish Ministry of Social Affairs and Health. (n.d.). History: From Grand Duchy to welfare state [Website]. https://stm.fi/en/ministry/history. Accessed 13 November 2019.
Frankford, D. M. (1994). Scientism and economism in the regulation of health care. *Journal of Health Politics, Policy and Law, 19*(4), 773–799.

Friel, S., & Marmot, M. (2011). Action on the social determinants of health and health inequities goes global. *Annual Review of Public Health, 32*, 225–236.

Glasgow, S. (2005). *The private life of public health: Managing chronic diseases in an era of neoliberal governmentality*. Ph.D. Thesis, University of Maryland.

Glasgow, S., & Schrecker, T. (2016). The double burden of neoliberalism? Noncommunicable disease policies and the global political economy of risk. *Health and Place., 39*, 204–211.

Glaze, S., & Richardson, B. (2017). Poor choice? Smith, Hayek and the moral economy of food consumption. *Economy and Society, 46*(1), 128–151.

Goldner Lang, I. (2017). Public health in European Union food law. In T. Hervey, C. Young, & L. Bishop (Eds.), *Research handbook on EU Health Law and Policy* (pp. 398–425). Edward Elgar.

Halpern, C., Jacquot, S., & Le Gales, P. (2014). *A mainstreaming: Analysis of a policy instrument* [Policy Brief]. NewGov: New Modes of Governance Project. HAL Archives Ouvertes.

Hammarström, A., & Ripper, M. (1999). What could a feminist perspective on power bring into public health? *Scandinavian Journal of Public Health., 27*, 286–289.

Hankivsky, O., & Christoffersen, A. (2008). Intersectionality and the determinants of health: A Canadian perspective. *Critical Public Health, 18*(3), 271–283.

Hawkes, C. (2005). The role of foreign direct investment in the nutrition transition. *Public Health Nutrition, 8*(4), 357–365.

Hawkes, C., Chopra, M., & Friel, S., et al. (2009). Globalization, trade and the nutrition transition. In R. Labonte, T. Schrecker, & C. Packer (Eds.), *Globalization and health: Pathways, evidence and policy* (pp. 235–262). Routledge.

Holder, H.D., Kühlhorn, E., Nordlund, S., Österberg, E., Romelsjö, A., & Ugland, T. (1998). *European integration and Nordic alcohol policies: Changes in alcohol controls and consequences in Finland, Norway and Sweden, 1980-97*. Routledge.

Horton, R. (2013). Non-communicable diseases: 2015 to 2025. *The Lancet, 381*(9866), 509–510.

Huynen, M., Martens, P., & Hilderink, H. (2005). The health impacts of globalisation: A conceptual framework. *Globalization and Health, 1*(14).

Jackson, T. (2018, December 23). *Paradise lost?—The iron cage of consumerism*. Centre for the Understanding of Sustainable Prosperity. https://cusp.ac.uk/themes/m/blog_tj_consumerism_as_theodicy/. Accessed 17 September 2012.

Jacquot, S. (2010). The paradox of gender mainstreaming: Unanticipated effects of new modes of governance in the gender equality domain. *West European Politics, 33*(1), 118–135.

Jarman, H., & Koivusalo, M. (2017). Trade and health in the European Union. In T. Hervey, C. Young, & L. Bishop (Eds.), *Research handbook on EU Health Law and Policy* (pp. 429–452). Edward Elgar.

Johns Hopkins Bloomberg School of Public Health. (n.d.). Leo Kaprio, MD, DrPH, MPH [Website]. https://www.jhsph.edu/about/history/heroes-of-public-health/leo-kaprio.html. Accessed 13 November 2019.

Jousilahti, P. (2014, September). *Health in All Policies – How was it achieved in Finland?* [PowerPoint presentation]. http://www.searo.who.int/entity/noncommunicable_diseases/events/ncd-bengaluru-health-in-all-policies-finland.pdf?ua=1. Accessed 11 November 2019.

Karanikolos, M., Mladovsky, P., Cylus, J., Thomson, S., Basu, S., Stuckler, D., Mackenbach, J. P., McKee, M. (2013). Financial crisis, austerity, and health in Europe. *The Lancet, 381*(9874), 1323–1331.

Kemm, J. (2001). Health impact assessment: A tool for Healthy Public Policy. *Health Promotion International, 16*(1), 79–85.

Kentikelenis, A., Karanikolos, M., Papanicolas, I., Basu, S., McKee, M., et al. (2011). Health effects of financial crisis: Omens of a Greek tragedy. *The Lancet, 378*(9801), 1457–1458.

Kickbusch, I. (1989). Approaches to an ecological base for public health. *Health Promotion, 4*(4), 265–268.

Kickbusch, I. (2003). The contribution of the World Health Organization to a new public health and health promotion. *American Journal of Public Health, 93*(3), 383–388.

Kickbusch, I., Williams, C., & Lawless, A. (2014). Making the most of open windows: Establishing Health in All Policies in South Australia. *International Journal of Health Services, 44*(1), 185–194.

Kingdon, J. W. (2014). *Agendas, alternative, and public policies* (2nd ed.). Pearson.

Knai, C., Petticrew, M., Capewell, S., Cassidy, R., Cummins, S., et al. (2018). Systems thinking as a framework for analyzing commercial determinants of health. *The Milbank Quarterly, 96*(3), 472–498.

Koivusalo, M. (2010). The state of Health in All Policies (HiAP) in the European Union: Potential and pitfalls. *Journal of Epidemiology and Community Health, 64*(6), 500–503.

Koivusalo, M. (2014). Policy space for health and trade and investment agreements. *Health Promotion International, 29*(Suppl. 1), i29-47.

Koivusalo, M., Heinonen, N., & Tynkkynen, L. (2021). When actions do not match aspirations - comparison of the European Union policy claims against what has been negotiated for health services, trade and investment. *Globalization and Health*. https://doi.org/10.1186/s12992-021-00739-8

Kokkinen, L., Muntaner, C., O'Campo, P., Freiler, A., Oneka, G., & Shankardass, K. (2019). Implementation of Health 2015 public health program in

Finland: A welfare state in transition. *Health Promotion International, 34*(2), 258–268.

Krieger, N. (2008). Proximal, distal, and the politics of causation: What's level got to do with it? *American Journal of Public Health, 98*(2), 221–230.

Labonté, R. (1998). Health promotion and the common good: Towards a politics of practice. *Critical Public Health, 8*(2), 107–129.

Labonté, R. (2014). Health in All (Foreign) Policies: Challenges in achieving coherence. *Health Promotion International, 29*(Suppl. 1), i48-58.

Labonté, R., & Schrecker, T. (2007a). Globalization and social determinants of health: Introduction and methodological background (Part 1 of 3). *Globalization and Health, 3*(5), 1–10.

Labonté, R., & Schrecker, T. (2007b). Globalization and social determinants of health: The role of the global marketplace (Part 2 of 3). *Globalization and Health, 3*(6), 1–17.

Labonté, R., & Schrecker, T. (2007c). Globalization and social determinants of health: Promoting health equity in global governance (Part 3 of 3). *Globalization and Health, 3*(7), 1–15.

Labonté, R., Mohindra, K., & Schrecker, T. (2011). The growing impact of globalization for Health and Public Health Practice. *Annual Review of Public Health, 32*, 263–283.

Lapalme, J., Haines-Saah, R., & Frohlich, K. L. (2019). More than a Buzzword: How Intersectionality Can Advance Social Inequalities in Health Research. *Critical Public Health* [Online]. https://doi.org/10.1080/09581596.2019.1584271

Lawn, J. E., Rohde, J., Rifkin, S., Were, M., Paul, V., et al. (2008). Alma-Ata 30 years on: Revolutionary, relevant, and time to revitalise. *The Lancet., 372*(9642), 917–927.

Lee, K., Sridhar, D., & Patel, M. (2009). Bridging the divide: Global governance of trade and health. *The Lancet, 373*(9661), 416–422.

Leppo, K., & Melkas, T. (1988). Towards healthy public policy: Experiences in Finland 1972–1987. *Health Promotion, 3*(2), 195–203.

Leppo, K., Ollila, E., Pena, S., Wismar, M., & Cook, S. (Eds.). (2013). *Health in All Policies: Seizing opportunities, implementing policies*. Ministry of Social Affairs and Health, Finland.

Lynch, J. (2020). *Regimes of inequality – The political economy of health and wealth*. Cambridge University Press.

Mackenbach, J. P. (2009). Politics is nothing but medicine at a larger scale: Reflections on public health's biggest idea. *Journal of Epidemiology and Community Health, 63*(3), 181–184.

Mahler, H. (1981). The meaning of 'health for all by the year 2000.' *World Health Forum, 2*(1), 5–22.

Marmot, M. (2005). Social determinants of health inequalities. *The Lancet, 365*(9464), 1099–1104.

Marmot, M. (2015). *The health gap*. Bloomsbury Publishing.

Marmot, M. (2018). Just societies, health equity, and dignified lives: The PAHO Equity Commission. *The Lancet, 392*(10161), 2247–2250.

Mauti, J., Gautier, L., De Neve, J., Beiersmann, C., Tosun, J., & Jahn, J. (2019). Kenya's Health in All Policies strategy: A policy analysis using Kingdon's multiple streams. *Health Research Policy and Systems, 17*(15).

McCartney, G., Collins, C., & Mackenzie, M. (2013). What (or who) causes health inequalities: Theories, evidence and implications? *Health Policy, 113*(3), 221–227.

McMahon, N. E. (2021). Working 'upstream' to reduce social inequalities in health: A qualitative study of how partners in an applied health research collaboration interpret the metaphor. *Critical Public Health*. https://doi.org/10.1080/09581596.2021.1931663

Melkas, T. (1988). Health for All by the Year 2000 – National finnish impact on the global development programme. *Scandinavian Journal of Social Medicine, 16*(1), 1–3.

Melkas, T. (2013). Health in All Policies as a priority in Finnish health policy: A case study on national health policy development. *Scandinavian Journal of Public Health, 41*(Suppl. 11), 3–28.

Merkel, B. (2010). *Health in All Policies 2010 – Dr. Bernard Merkel* [Video uploaded on Vimeo]. *SA Health Conference, Government of South Australia*. https://vimeo.com/13389841. Accessed 13 November 2019.

Mialon, M. (2020). An overview of the commercial determinants of health. *Globalization and Health, 16*(74). https://doi.org/10.1186/s12992-020-00607-x

Mikkonen, J. (2018). *Intersectoral action for health: Challenges, opportunities, and future directions in the WHO European Region*. Ph.D. Thesis, York University, Toronto.

Mittelmark, M. B., Sagy, S., Eriksson, M., Bauer, G. F., Pelikan, J. M., Lindström, B., Vaandrager, L., & Magistretti, C. M. (Eds.). (2017). *The handbook of Salutogenesis* [Open Access eBook]: Springer.

Navarro, V., & Shi, L. (2001). The political context of social inequalities and health. *International Journal of Health Services, 31*(1), 1–21.

Navarro, V., Muntaner, C., Borrell, C., Benach, J., Quiroga, A., Rodríguez-Sanz, M., Vergés, N., & Pasarín, M. I. (2006). Politics and health outcomes. *The Lancet, 368*(9540), 1033–1037.

Nousianen, P. (2018). Municipal self-governance. In: I. Taipale (Ed.), *100 social innovations from Finland* (pp. 28–30). Leo Mechelin Foundation.

Ollila, E. (2011). Health in All Policies: From rhetoric to action. *Scandinavian Journal of Public Health, 39*(Suppl. 6), 11–18.

Ollila, E., Ståhl, T., Wismar, M., Lahtinen, E., Melkas, T., Melkas, T., & Leppo, K. (2006). *Health in All Policies in the European Union and its member states* [Policy Brief]. https://ec.europa.eu/health/ph_projects/2005/action1/docs/2005_1_18_frep_a4_en.pdf. Accessed 11 November 2019.

Oneka, G., Vahid Shahidi, F., Muntaner, C., Bayoumi, A. M., Mahabir, D. F., et al. (2017). A glossary of terms for understanding political aspects in the implementation of Health in All Policies (HiAP). *Journal of Epidemiology and Community Health, 71*(8), 835–838.

Ottersen, O. P., Dasgupta, J., Blouin, C., Buss, P., Chongsuvivatwong, V., et al. (2014). The political origins of health inequity: Prospects for change. *The Lancet, 383*(9917), 630–667.

Paradies, Y. (2016). Colonisation, racism and indigenous health. *Journal of Population Research, 33*, 83–96.

Parkhurst, J. (2017). *The politics of evidence: From evidence-based policy to the good governance of evidence*. Routledge.

Peck, J., & Tickell, A. (2002). Neoliberalizing space. *Antipode, 34*(3), 380–404.

Peck, J., & Tickell, A. (2007). Conceptualizing neoliberalism, thinking Thatcherism. In H. Leitner, J. Peck, & E. S. Sheppard (Eds.), *Contesting neoliberalism: Urban frontiers* (pp. 26–50). The Guilford Press.

Pollack, M. A., & Hafner-Burton, E. (2000). Mainstreaming gender in the European Union. *Journal of European Public Policy, 7*(3), 432–456.

Putnam, S., & Galea, S. (2008). Epidemiology and the macrosocial determinants of health. *Journal of Public Health Policy, 29*, 275–289.

Rose, N., O'Malley, P., & Valverde, M. (2006). Governmentality. *Annual Review of Law and Social Science, 2*, 83–104.

Rogers, W. A. (2006). Feminism and public health ethics. *Journal of Medical Ethics, 32*, 351–354.

Rouvinen-Wilenius, P., Ahokas, J., Kiukas, V., & Aalto-Kallio, M. (2019). Finnish NGOs promoting health equity in the context of welfare economy. *Health Promotion International, 34*(4), 648–657.

Sacco, R. L., Smith, S. C., Holmes, D., Shurin, S., Brawley, O., Cazap, E., Glass, R., Komajda, M., Koroshetz, W., Mayer-Davis, E., Mbanya, J. C., Sledge, G., & Varmus, H. (2013). Accelerating progress on non-communicable diseases. *The Lancet, 382*(9895), e4–e5.

Sadler, D., & Lloyd, S. (2009). Neo-liberalising corporate social responsibility: A political economy of corporate citizenship [Online article]. *Geoforum*. https://doi.org/10.1016/j.geoforum.2009.03.008

Schorb, F. (2013). Fat politics in Europe: Theorizing on the premises and outcomes of European Anti-"obesity-Epidemic" policies. *Fat Studies, 2*(1), 3–16.

Schrecker, T., & Bambra, C. (2015). *How Politics makes us sick: Neoliberal epidemics*. Palgrave Macmillan.

Sell, S. K., & Williams, O. D. (2020). Health under capitalism: A global political economy of structural pathogenesis. *Review of International Political Economy, 27*(1), 1–25.

Shankardass, K., Muntaner, C., Kokkinen, L., Vahid Shahidi, F., Freiler, A., Freiler, A., Oneka, G., Bayoumi, A. M., & O'Campo, P. (2018). The implementation of Health in All Policies initiatives: A systems framework for government action. *Health Research Policy and Systems, 16*(26), 1–10.

Sheldon, T. A., & Wright, J. (2020). Twin epidemics of covid-19 and non-communicable disease. *BMJ Editorial*. https://doi.org/10.1136/bmj.m2618

Smith, K. E. (2013). *Beyond evidence-based policy in public health: The interplay of ideas*. Palgrave Macmillan.

Sparke, M. (2016). Health and the embodiment of neoliberalism: Pathologies of political economy from climate change and austerity to personal responsibility. In S. Springer, K. Birch, & J. MacLeavy (Eds.), *The handbook of neoliberalism* (pp. 237–252). Routledge.

Sparke, M. (2020). Neoliberal regime change and the remaking of global health: From rollback disinvestment to rollout reinvestment and reterritorialization. *Review of International Political Economy, 27*(1), 48–74.

Ståhl, T., & Lahtinen, E. (2006). Towards closer intersectoral cooperation: The preparation of the Finnish national health report. In T. Ståhl, M. Wismar, E. Ollila, Lahtinen E., & Leppo, K. (Eds.), *Health in All Policies: Prospect and potentials* (pp. 169–185). Helsinki: Ministry of Social Affairs and Health, Finland.

Ståhl, T., Wismar, M., Ollila, E., Lahtinen, E., & Leppo, K. (Eds.). (2006). *Health in All Policies: Prospects and potentials*. Ministry of Social Affairs and Health, Finland.

Stuckler, D., & Basu, S. (2013). *The body economics: Why Austerity kills*. Basic Books.

Stuckler, D., Basu, S., & McKee, M. (2010). Budget crises, health, and social welfare programmes. *BMJ, 340*(c:3311), 77–79.

Stuckler, D., Reeves, A., Loopstra, R., Karanikolos, M., & McKee, M. (2017). Austerity and health: The impact in the UK and Europe. *European Journal of Public Health, 27*(Suppl. 4), 18–21.

Synnevåg, E. S., Amdam, R., & Fosse, E. (2018). Public health terminology: Hindrance to a Health in All Policies approach? *Scandinavian Journal of Public Health, 46*(1), 68–73.

Taipale, I. (2018). *100 social innovations from Finland*. Leo Mechelin Foundation.

Taipale, V. (2002). Challenges in health promotion policies. *IUHPE – Promotion & Education, 9*(4), 143–146.

Tang., K. C., Ståhl, T., Bettcher, D., De Leeuw, E. (2014). The Eighth Global Conference on Health Promotion: Health in All Policies – From rhetoric to action. *Health Promotion International, 29*(Suppl. 1), i1–i8.

The Lancet (Editorial), (2020). COVID-19: A new lens for non-communicable diseases. *The Lancet*. https://doi.org/10.1016/%20S0140-6736(20)31761-X

Thorsen, D. E., & Lie, A. (2006). *What is neoliberalism?* (Working Paper). Department of Political Science, University of Oslo. http://folk.uio.no/daget/What%20is%20Neo-Liberalism%20FINAL.pdf. Accessed 11 November 2019.

Townsend, P., Davidson, N., & Whitehead, M. (1992). *Inequalities in health: The black report and the health divide*. Penguin.

True, J. (2003). Mainstreaming gender in global public policy. *International Feminist Journal of Politics, 5*(3), 368–396.

Van den Broucke, S. (2014). Needs, norms and nudges: The place of behaviour change in health promotion. *Health Promotion International, 29*(4), 597–600.

Vander, C. (2007). The politics of health as a school-sponsored ethic. *Educational Policy, 22*(6), 854–874.

Vander Schee, C. (2009). Fruit, vegetables, fatness, and Foucault: Governing students and their families through school health policy. *Journal of Education Policy, 24*(5), 557–574.

Verloo, M. (2005). Mainstreaming Gender Equality in Europe. A Critical Frame Analysis Approach. *The Greek Review of Social Research, 117*, 11–34.

Virtanen, T., et al. (2016). Finland: Active Reformer looking for more centralisation and horizontal coordination. In G. Hammerschmid, R. Van der Walle, & R. Andrews (Eds.), *Public administration reforms in Europe: The view from the top* (pp. 129–139). Edward Elgar.

Watts, N., Amann, M., Ayeb-Karlsson, S., Belesova, K., Bouley, T., Boykoff, M., Byass, P., Cai, W., Campbell-Lendrum, D., Chambers, J., Cox, P. M., Daly, M., Dasandi, N., Davies, M., Depledge, M., Depoux, A., Dominguez-Salas, P., Drummond, P., Ekins, P., et al. (2018). The Lancet Countdown on health and climate change: From 25 years of inaction to a global transformation for public health. *The Lancet, 391*, 581–630.

Whitehead, M. (1991). The concept and principles of equity and health. *Health Promotion International, 6*(3), 217–228.

WHO. (1978). *Declaration of Alma Ata*. International Conference of Primary Health Care. https://www.who.int/publications/almaata_declaration_en.pdf. Accessed 11 September 2019.

WHO. (1981). *Global Strategy for health for all by the year 2000*. https://iris.wpro.who.int/bitstream/handle/10665.1/6967/WPR_RC032_GlobalStrategy_1981_en.pdf. Accessed 11 September 2019.

WHO. (1986). *Ottawa Charter for health promotion.* http://www.euro.who.int/__data/assets/pdf_file/0004/129532/Ottawa_Charter.pdf. Accessed 18 November 2019.

WHO. (2008). *Closing the gap in a generation: Health equity through action on the social determinants of health.* WHO Commission on Social Determinants of health, Final Report.

WHO. (2013). The Helsinki Statement. *Health Promotion International, 29*(Suppl. 1), i17–i18.

WHO. (2014a). Health in All Policies (HiAP) Framework for Country Action. *Health Promotion International*, Vol 29. *Supplement, 1*, i19–i28.

WHO. (2014b). What you need to know about Health in All Policies. *World Health Organization, 36*(1), 20–21.

WHO.(2015a). *Finland curbs childhood obesity by integrating Health in All Policies* [Website]. https://www.who.int/features/2015/finland-health-in-all-policies/en/. Accessed 11 September 2019.

WHO. (2015b). *Health in All Policies: Training manual.* https://apps.who.int/iris/bitstream/handle/10665/151788/9789241507981_eng.pdf;jsessionid=1C51E025953B98A18AE5F70DAAD49F86?sequence=1. Accessed 11 September 2019.

WHO. (2015c). *Finland: How to take into account Health, Wellbeing and Equity in all sectors in Finland* [Country cases studies on Primary Healthcare]. Accessed 17 September 2019.

WHO. (2018a, June 1). *Noncommunicable diseases – Key facts* [Website]. https://www.who.int/news-room/fact-sheets/detail/noncommunicable-diseases. Accessed 13 November 2019.

WHO, (2018b). *Key learning on Health in All Policies implementation from around the world information brochure.* https://apps.who.int/iris/bitstream/handle/10665/272711/WHO-CED-PHE-SDH-18.1-eng.pdf?ua=1. Accessed 11 September 2019.

Wilkinson, R. G., & Pickett, K. (2010). *The spirit level: Why equality is better for everyone* (2nd ed.). Penguin Books.

Wilkinson, R. G., & Pickett, K. (2018). *The inner level: How more equal societies reduce stress, restore sanity and improve everyone's well-being.* Penguin Books.

Zinsstag, J., Schelling, E., Waltner-Toews, D., & Tanner, M. (2011). From 'one medicine' to 'one health' and systemic approaches to health and well-being. *Preventive Veterinary Medicine, 101*(3–4), 148–156.

Zuccala, E., & Horton, R. (2020). Reframing the NCD agenda: A matter of justice and equity. *The Lancet Comment.* https://doi.org/10.1016/

CHAPTER 3

Where Is 'Health' in EU Governance?

The discussion around macrosocial determinants of health suggests that, even if public health per se is largely a member state competence, EU competencies still influence it. But how should we navigate this massive entity that is the EU, to identify its relevance to HiAP? This book does not provide an exhaustive account of all policy areas directly and indirectly relevant to health—such a task would be monumental. Instead, it is concerned with studying HiAP as a soft, cognitive process requiring an approach focused on meaning-making (Jacquot, 2010). Still, some form of navigation map is required, which is what this chapter provides. It builds on existing research and outlines a categorisation of EU governance types: soft, hard and meta-regulatory governance, along which the scope for HiAP will be studied. Most research critically looking at the politics of health in the EU focuses on health(care) policy and law, and critiques the constitutionally asymmetrical integration dynamics that privilege markets over people (Greer, 2014a; Greer & Löblová, 2016; Lamping & Steffen, 2009). While sympathetic to these points, this chapter sets the scene for taking this critique a step further by considering macrosocial determinants of health. This arguably broadens the scope of EU health studies.

C. Godziewski, *The Politics of Health Promotion*, Palgrave Studies in Science, Knowledge and Policy, https://doi.org/10.1007/978-3-030-97870-9_3

3.1 EU Integration and the Growing Involvement in Public Health

Before telling the story of the EU's involvement in public health, let's start with a short introduction to the EU institutions, as well as to how EU integration has been theorised. The EU's functions are legally based on treaties, a series of which were signed over the decades. To get a sense of how EU governance relates to health, it is worth mentioning two treaties in particular: the Maastricht Treaty, signed in 1992, and the Lisbon Treaty in 2007. The Maastricht Treaty is the initial Treaty of the European Union, which established three pillars of the EU: the European Communities, the Common Foreign and Security Policy, and cooperation in the fields of Justice and Home Affairs (Bache et al., 2015). The Maastricht Treaty considerably furthered European integration, notably by establishing the European Monetary Union (EMU). EMU relates to the creation of the Eurozone, the creation of the Euro as a common currency, and the Stability and Growth Pact (SGP). It is because of EMU that, later down the line (especially after the Eurozone crisis), the EU became increasingly involved in member states' fiscal policies. Maastricht also expanded the EU competencies in many social areas, including health and public health, even though this was not done through the same pathways as the expansion of economic competencies. The Lisbon Treaty is the most recently signed EU treaty. The Lisbon Treaty did not consolidate all previous treaties into one constitution, as was originally hoped (and originally planned to be named the 'Constitutional Treaty'). Instead, it kept the two-treaty structure[1] put in place in 1997, but with a considerable number of amendments. These two treaties are: the Treaty of the European Union (TEU) and the Treaty on the Functioning of the European Union (TFEU, formerly known as the Treaty of the European Community, 'TEC'). The TEU comprises aspects related to overarching principles of the EU, such as the conditions and processes for accession and withdrawal, the EU's broad principles, its institutional makeup, as well as matter related to the Common Foreign and Security Policy. The TFEU, on the other hand, governs every aspect of the actual functioning of the EU, also referred to as 'the Union Method' (EUR-Lex, 2010).

The TFEU establishes the level of EU 'competence', which dictates how much the EU is mandated to do in a particular area. Some areas are

[1] A third treaty not mentioned here is the Euratom Treaty.

exclusive EU competence, many areas are shared competencies, and in some areas, the EU only has supportive competence (European Union, 2016). These competencies are subject to three fundamental principles: the principle of conferral, which states that the competencies are conferred to the EU by the member states; the principle of proportionality, which states that in the exercise of its competencies, the EU should not go beyond what is necessary to achieve a set objective; and finally, the principle of subsidiarity, which states that, in non-exclusive EU competencies, decision-making and action taking should occur at EU level only if the EU member states are not able to achieve a set objective on their own (priority is given to the governance level closest to the citizens) (European Union, 2016).

The EC is (arguably) the most important institution when analysing EU level governance. Its two biggest responsibilities are proposing legislation and drafting the EU budget (Staab, 2013). The EC is also responsible for ensuring the appropriate enactment of EU legislation by member states. If the EC or another entity (another member state or even a citizen) finds that a member state is breaking EU law, the case can be handled by the Court of Justice of the European Union (CJEU). The EC works with executive agencies, such as, in the area of health, the European Centre for Disease Control (ECDC), the European Medicines Agency (EMA) and the Consumer, Health, Agriculture and Food Executive Agency (CHAFEA). In addition to the EC, the European Council also has non-negligible agenda-setting powers (Bache et al., 2015, p. 204). The European Council is composed of the heads of member states, the EC president and a high representative for foreign and security policy. In terms of agenda-setting powers, the EP also has the possibility to request the EC to submit a legislative proposal under certain conditions. The EP and the Council of Ministers (normally referred to as 'the Council', as opposed to 'the European Council') are the bodies that vote on EC proposals. Once a legislative proposal has been drafted, it goes to both the Council and the EP for a 'co-decision' process. The Council is officially composed of member states ministers, but in practice it works through committees of member states' officials. The Council and the EP vote on an EC proposal either by unanimity, by qualified majority voting, or by 'reversed qualified majority', depending on the situation. The EP consists of elected members and comprises several committees.

A classic debate in EU academic literature pertains to seeing the EU as either an intergovernmental institution or a supranational institution

(Pollack, 2001). According to neofunctionalist theory, European integration occurs through various kinds of 'spill over'. This refers to how integrating in one area induces the need to expand integration beyond that area, because of knock-on effects and path dependencies (Haas, 1958). Besides functional ('automatic') spill over, neofunctionalists argue that spill over can also be intentionally cultivated by interest group who see a benefit in bypassing the national level. Additionally, and in interaction with interests groups, spill over is also pushed by the so-called socialised elites consisting of supranational civil servant who have been socialised into favouring supranational (in this case, EU level) solutions (Jensen, 2009; Niemann & Ioannou, 2015). Quite a few EU health scholars have drawn on these neofunctionalist concepts to explain the growing involvement of the EU in health policy and law (Greer, 2006; Greer & Löblová, 2016). Though unlike many neofunctionalists, they question the legitimacy and desirability of further integration, rather than taking it as desirable by default. For long, neofunctionalist theory of EU integration stood in binary opposition to the 'intergovernmentalist' theorisation of EU integration. Arguably, the most sophisticated intergovernmentalist branch is liberal intergovernmentalism, according to which integration results from bargaining processes of rational-acting states and occurs along the lowest denominator when economic interests converge (Cini, 2009; Moravcsik, 1998).

This (simplified) binary opposition between intergovernmentalism and neofunctionalism characterises much of the early-day (and to an extent still enduring) EU integration debates which draw on IR theories. The last few decades, however, have been marked by a shift towards other ways to look at the EU. These 'newer' theories are more concerned with analysing the EU from a governance angle, looking to explain specific parts of the EU and avoiding 'grand theories' angles that characterise the IR approach (Rosamond, 2009, p. 108). Arguably, this reflects a shift in interest away from identifying the drivers of integration and towards understanding the workings of the EU. For example, multi-level governance approaches, and policymaking theories of the EU in general, contest the idea of a clear distinction between national and EU (and international) levels (Bache & Flinders, 2004). They focus on the intricacies of policymaking as processes determined by complex networked structures. Variants of 'new institutionalism' also reflect the governance turn in EU studies, as they put the accent on the role of institutions, which they define in different ways. Constructivist theories have also increasingly been applied to the EU (see, for example, Parker, 2018; Parker & Pye, 2018; Radaelli, 2007; Rosamond, 2002; Siles-Brügge, 2013). We will come back to this in the next chapter.

Constitutional Asymmetry

One concept derived from EU integration theory and important for the purposes of this book is the notion of 'constitutional asymmetry' (Scharpf, 2002). The EU integration process and the institutional expansion over the decades did not happen in a smooth linear fashion, but rather with various episodes of bursts and pushbacks. The EU project at its root, however, can be seen as an economic project of market integration aimed at the social goal of peace and prosperity promotion. After two world wars, the six founding members were ready to negotiate aspects of their national sovereignty in order to promote peace and unity (Bache et al., 2015). At the same time, the Marshall Plan provided the impetus to foster economic cooperation between European countries (Staab, 2013). The initial rationale for economic integration was that pooling the market of steel and coal and increasing interdependency for the provision of these resources would decrease the likelihood of another war (Bache et al., 2015). As a result of these historical and contingent developments, the EU became much better equipped to regulate economic matters, than to get involved in social areas. One aspect to consider is that the EU is inherently a regulatory polity with very little redistributive power (Majone, 1993, 2014). The EU, for example, does not collect taxes. Its budget, proportionally speaking, is very small, around one percent of member states' gross national income. The EU also has generally limited competencies in regulating social areas. What dominates in the EU is the power to regulate economic areas, such as Single Market integration and EMU. The term 'constitutional asymmetry' encapsulates these differential integration dynamics. It refers to the disproportionate weight given to economic policies and the ease of their integration, compared to social policies. This is reflected in the treaties, in the legal competencies and procedures in place (Greer et al., 2014).

While the EU project was primarily one of economic integration, expectations to strengthen its 'social logics' started intensifying as economic integration became deep enough for legal constraints on domestic welfare states to be felt (Scharpf, 2002). 'Negative integration', which acts to remove barriers to trade and promote the freedom of the Single Market, tends to be systematically stronger and faster than 'positive' (i.e. market correcting) forms of integration (Scharpf, 1998). Because of the executive power of the EC and the authority of the CJEU, negative integration becomes depoliticised, whereas positive integration needs political legitimation and a high level of consensus. This is often hard to achieve due to strongly varying interests and modes of welfare governance of member states (Scharpf, 2006). Relatedly, Scharpf explains that, while 'product-related regulation' guaranteeing quality and safety standards has been fairly easy to put in place alongside negative integration, 'process-related regulation' at EU level, such as those pertaining to labour rights, is not easily justifiable and agreed upon because they do not directly determine the safety and quality of the end product in the market (Scharpf, 1997, 2006). In the case of health promotion, this rationale is illustrated in the importance given to food safety and sanitary and phytosanitary (SPS) regulations, as opposed to action on macrosocial determinants of NCDs—despite NCDs being the biggest burden of disease in the EU. The relative ease of negative integration compared to positive integration is symptomatic of the existing constitutional asymmetry and is the reason why some researchers argue that the EU presents an institutionally ingrained *neoliberal* bias (Bailey, 2017; Gill, 1998; van Apeldoorn et al., 2009; Walters & Haahr, 2005).

With those theoretical considerations in mind, let us now turn to the story of the EU's growing involvement in health, up until the end of the Juncker EC presidency in November 2019. Technically, the EU only has shared competence for 'shared safety concerns in public health matters', and only supportive competencies for 'protection and improvement of human health' (European Union, 2016, pp. 1–2). At first sight, one might thus question the legitimacy of EU health governance even as a research subject, given the limited competence. In practice, however, the EU has been having a tremendous effect on the population's health, in terms of both public health and individual healthcare, in several different ways (Steffen et al., 2005). Officially, the involvement of the EU in health is categorised under three pillars: healthcare policy, public health and occupational health and safety policy (Anderson, 2015). The first one is not directly related to health promotion, as it refers to curative services related to a medical definition of health: access, administration and financing of health services (hospitals and medical offices, medicines and medical devices, and health insurance). Public health policy, in the EU literature, refers in the largest part to the control and surveillance of communicable diseases, including foodborne diseases, as well as food safety more generally. The first health-specific legislation, for example, was the directive on colourant in foodstuffs and was adopted in 1962 (Guy & Sauter, 2017). The continued emphasis on food safety is in part due to the story of the EU involvement in public health being very closely linked to the outbreak of mad cow disease in the late 1990s. Indeed, the EC's DG concerned with health was not set up 'as its own DG', but emerged as an enhancement of the DG for consumer protection, at the time of health and food safety concerns related to the mad cow disease crisis (Clemens et al., 2017; Geyer & Lightfoot, 2010). At that time, it was called DG SANCO, for health, food safety and consumer protection, whereas now the DG for health is called DG SANTE and oversees health and food safety. Environmental health and, to a smaller extent, the promotion of healthy behaviours are also included under the EU public health category. Finally, occupational health and safety is the third category which characterises the EU's involvement in health. This one is also of historical significance because it pertains to workers' rights and freedom of movement of labour. The first health-related provision was adopted as early as 1958 and pertained to the free movement of workers in the EU and social security coordination (Guy & Sauter, 2017).

The TFEU includes one specific public health article: Article 168. It states, among other things, that the EU has a responsibility to take into consideration and strive to improve the health of its citizens through every action it undertakes. The breadth of the article makes it compellingly strong, but its vagueness undermines this strength, as defining what promoting and safeguarding health refers to is political.

The way in which the EU got involved in health policy and law was in an incremental, ad hoc fashion, which may now explain the 'patchwork' or 'Christmas tree' condition of EU health law and policy: its involvement in health did not stem from a coherent, comprehensive strategy, but happened largely through a Single Market harmonisation rationale (Lamping & Steffen, 2009). Indeed, critical EU health scholars often draw on the concept of spill over, in the context of asymmetrical integration favouring economic over social integration, to make sense of the EU's involvement in health (Greer, 2006, 2014a, Greer & Löblová, 2016; Lamping, 2005; Lamping & Steffen, 2009). EU involvement in health policy is seen to result from interest groups dissatisfied at their national-level governments and turning towards the EU, ultimately conferring upon it the legitimacy to act on one particular issue and leading to an ever-growing area of EU action related to that issue (Greer, 2009). As Greer (2009, p. 4) puts it: 'The whole problem of EU health policy is that most of the policies enter from adjacent fields rather than health ministers or health agendas'.

The CJEU's interpretation of internal market legislation played a larger role in shaping EU health policies and law, than competencies in health per se (Anderson, 2015; Mossialos et al., 2010; Sindbjerg Martinsen, 2017; de Ruijiter, 2019). The case of cross-border patient mobility illustrates the prominent—yet not unchallengeable—role of the CJEU and spill over effects (Brooks, 2012). Alcohol policy is another example of the CJEU's tendency to prioritise negative, market-creating integration over public health (though portraying this as an all-or-nothing situation would be an oversimplification) (Baumberg & Andersen, 2008).

'Three Faces' of EU Involvement in Health

In light of the asymmetric logics of EU integration systematically favouring markets over social issues, Scott Greer has categorised the involvement of the EU in health under three 'faces' (Greer, 2014a). He argues that, in line with the constitutionally asymmetric nature of EU institutions, the EU's involvement in health is driven mostly by non-health rationales. This is reflected by the avenues for health laws and policies lying largely *outside* the health policy field. This results in a market logic becoming imposed in areas that, like health, are situated in the social sphere. Policies designed purely with a public health goal in mind represent a very small minority of EU involvement in health. This, he classifies as the 'first face' of EU involvement in health, in contrast to the second face (Single Market integration) and the third face (fiscal coordination) of EU involvement in health.

Given the limited competencies in health, first-face involvement tends to be non-binding support for member state. This is largely the case in NCD prevention and health promotion. Garde (2010) points out that the development of an EU competence in obesity-related issues is limited to a supportive, non-binding role and translates into two main ways: one is the funding of public health research, and the other pertains to the coordination, evaluation, monitoring and advising of member states (Garde, 2010). Second-face involvement occurs through Single Market integration. This is arguably the most developed avenue for EU involvement in health and is generally more binding. Single Market regulations have implications for the free movement of healthcare-related goods, services and patient and health workforce mobility. Food safety is ensured through Single Market laws, for example, by ensuring common SPS standards. Some emblematic examples of EU health involvement through the Single Market include the directives regulating the handling of human blood, tissue and cells (European Union, 2003, 2004b), or the directive relating to patients' mobility (European Union, 2011). The latter explicitly shows how the internal market serves as a treaty basis despite the public health relevance of the directive:

> Article 114 TFEU [*i.e. the Article pertaining to the governance of the Single Market*] is the appropriate legal basis since the majority of the provisions of this Directive aim to improve the functioning of the internal market and the free movement of goods, persons and services. Given that the conditions for recourse to Article 114 TFEU as a legal basis are fulfilled, Union legislation has to rely on this legal basis even when public health protection is a decisive factor in the choices made. (European Union, 2011, p. 45)

The newest, third-face action pertains to EU economic and fiscal coordination (Fahy, 2012; Greer, 2014b). This avenue for involvement in health policy and law emerged because of the Eurozone crisis and the toughening of fiscal coordination between member states. The EU's involvement in member states' fiscal governance has direct implications for national health systems, which are pushed towards more cost-effectiveness and modernisation/digitalisation. The impact on member states' health systems of these relatively new coordination tools, such as the European Semester for example, is increasingly researched (Azzopardi-Muscat et al., 2015; Greer, 2014a).

In sum, one common way to critically conceptualise the EU's involvement in health is to see it as resulting from some form of spill over in the context of asymmetrical integration dynamics that favour freedom of market over social protection.[2] In that sense, the EU involvement in health policy and law represents an illegitimate encroachment, 'uninvited Europeanization' (Greer, 2006) that crept in through the backdoor of the

[2] One notably different approach is taken by Flear (2015), who uses a Foucauldian, biopolitical framework to critically analyse EU health policy.

CJEU and the EC (Anderson, 2015; Liebfried, 2010). Indeed, if health concerns are not even the main driver for most involvement of the EU in health, and if the public health article of the TFEU (Article 168) is hardly an important legal basis for most EU involvement in health, what does that say about the nature of involvement in health?

> Health is a perfect case of European integration – negative, deregulating integration – driven by the EU institutions without democratic legitimacy or an obvious justification. It is driven by EU institutions and produces markets where there were none, in order to make systems compatible with the EU internal market. (Greer, 2014a, p. 11)

This book is sympathetic to these arguments; indeed, it concurs with and draws on them (particularly in Chapter 5). However, one suggestion this book makes is that the relationship between the EU, neoliberal rationality, and health should be conceptualised both more broadly and in a more nuanced, less deterministic way. By focusing on healthcare and health systems, we neglect the crucial role of (macrosocial) determinants of health and health promotion, which are not necessarily shaped by health policies and health laws. Relatedly, a broader conceptualisation of the relationship between neoliberalism, the EU and health also needs to pay more attention to the effects of soft governance. Softer, less binding ways to govern need to be taken seriously when critiquing the infusion of a market rationality in social areas. While much of the critical literature on the EU and health eloquently demonstrates how the increasing involvement of the EU in health is underpinned by a market rationality, it is arguably not concerned enough with the notion of neoliberalism itself, the various dynamics of how it manifests and the multiplicity of ways in which it affects health.

Rather than showing that a concern for economic growth and market creation drives the EU's increasing involvement in health policy and law, this book starts with the notion of HiAP to consider the more general effects of neoliberalism on population health, whether manifested in health policy or in entirely different policies. Instead of being concerned solely with the EU neoliberal intrusion into health policy and health systems, it is concerned with how neoliberalism is reproduced more broadly, and how that affects the possibility to consider health in other policy areas. Implementing HiAP, in that sense, would need to entail a move away from neoliberal governance. Of course, one might ask: 'if even

EU health policies are not about health, then how could EU non-health policies be about health?'. This is where the need for more nuance comes in. While this book recognises the issues of constitutional asymmetry and EU neoliberal biases, it rejects the idea of the EU as a pre-determined neoliberal monolith. The very point that HiAP did make it to the EU agenda suggests that the way these institutions evolve is not *homogenously* neoliberal.

A concern with HiAP at EU level, then, also feeds into the debates around social versus economic EU, and how to make Europe more social (Ferrera, 2017; van Gerven & Ossewaarde, 2018), only the lens used here to look at the social sphere, is health and the macrosocial determinants of health. This is a highly relevant focus to be taking, as it is likely to grow in importance in the aftermath of the coronavirus pandemic.

3.2 Mapping the Territory

Studying a concept that is supposed to be mainstreamed across the board inevitably means covering a lot of ground empirically. This is even more considerable as we are using a very broad definition of health, health promotion and determinants of health. To navigate this large scope, I will clarify along which dimensions EU governance areas will be categorised: hard governance, soft governance and meta-regulatory governance. The differentiation between 'hard' and 'soft' EU governance is widely drawn upon and relates to Scharpf's concepts of negative and positive integration, and constitutional asymmetry (Greer, 2014a). The hard/soft divide also fits well with the three-face categorisation of involvement in health. In addition to the soft/hard divide, I point out the importance of a third category, especially as HiAP pertains to a cognitive mainstreaming exercise: meta-regulatory governance (Radaelli, 2007). While the three-face categorisation is very useful and particularly well adapted to studying healthcare-related policy in the EU, it does not entirely fit in a context of studying HiAP. Studying HiAP in the EU is not so much about 'how do non-health EU competencies spill over into the health sector and in turn affect health', but more about 'how do non-health EU competencies affect macrosocial determinants of population health themselves'. It then becomes necessary to go beyond the three-face categorisation that considers only soft and hard governance styles, to also look at the EU meta-regulatory agenda (Table 3.1).

Table 3.1 Examples of EU governance areas by EU governance type

Hard governance	*Soft governance*	*Meta-regulatory governance*
• The Single European Market • European fiscal governance: the SGP reforms	• New Modes of Governance	• The Better Regulation Agenda • The collegiality principle

Bearing these three categories in mind will guide us through the rest of the book. Even though I will argue for the need to look beyond the soft/hard dichotomy, the soft/hard/meta-classification is nevertheless a useful notion to orient oneself within the EU governance sphere: Chapter 5 follows the soft/hard/meta-classification quite closely, whereas Chapters 6 and 7 will demonstrate the need to also consider ideational and discursive forms of power.

'Hard' Governance

Hard governance refers mostly to EU exclusive (and shared) competencies and any areas of EU governance in which the EU exerts power, in a legally-binding, sanctionable way. Examples of hard governance introduced here are Single Market integration and European fiscal governance (especially since the Eurozone crisis). Both these areas mostly pertain to economic governance as opposed to social governance—even though arguably the European Semester can be seen as a link between the two.

One of the main aspects of EU integration has been the drive to create a single European market. This started with the creation of a customs union and the gradual removal of tariff barriers, and later also non-tariff barriers, between member states. The idea of a Single Market is associated with the famous 'indivisible four freedoms' principle enshrined the treaties: freedom of movement of goods, services, capital and labour. Under the Juncker Commission, DG GROW was the DG responsible for the internal market, industry, entrepreneurship and SMEs. Its task is to integrate the Single Market and remove barriers to trade. It aims to unleash 'the full potential' of EU businesses and offer more choice and freedom to consumers, while promoting economic growth. Proponents of the Single Market emphasise how high consumer protection standards have allowed the Single Market to increase consumer choice, lower prices while safeguarding safety and quality standards (including in food safety), making those standards the EU market distinctive brand (European Parliament, 2018). The 'hard', binding instruments at the disposal of the EU for pushing Single Market integration are mostly regulations and directives. Regulations are directly applicable, whereas directives need to be transposed into national legislation (European Union, 2004a).

Some have pointed out pressures from the EU to open up and liberalise national services such as healthcare and public transport among other things (Buch-Hansen & Wigger, 2010; Hall, 2002; Héritier, 2001; Van Apeldoorn & Horn, 2018). The Single Market has also been criticised for challenging national public health policies deemed unfair trade barriers, notably alcohol policies in Nordic countries. Many Single Market-related acts are directives, which means they set out a goal, and member states are free to decide how they will transpose it into national legislation. This can give considerable discretion in interpreting and implementing Single Market policies. *Some* of those member states generally reluctant to embrace neoliberal governance have been broadly able to protect their national services from 'wild' deregulation,[3] albeit not without hard work and negotiation (Melkas, 2013). A newer aspect of the Single Market which is growing in importance since the Juncker Commission is the 'Digital' Single Market. The idea of the Digital Single Market is to boost and remove barriers to e-commerce within the EU, jumping on the big data analytics bandwagon, improving digital facilities and improving consumer data protection (European Commission, 2015a).

The EU also adopts a 'hard' governance stance when it comes to the coordination of the economic and monetary union of the EU, especially since the Eurozone crisis. If the initial EU project was about creating a Single Market and removing barriers to the free movement of capital, goods, services and people within that market, the creation of the EMU has increasingly developed an important additional area of integration and coordination. The stronger interdependence between member states resulting from the EMU led to the adoption of the SGP. The purpose of the SGP is to ensure all member states aim to keep their national debt and deficit below a certain threshold, to ensure the stability and economic

[3] While this may be the case for the Nordic member states, it is not necessarily so for Mediterranean countries most affected by the crisis (see Greer, 2014b).

convergence of member states. After the Eurozone crisis, (some) member states decided the mechanisms to ensure compliance with the SGP should be tightened. This led to the so-called six-pack and two-pack reforms of 2011 and 2013. These reforms consist of a set of preventive and corrective binding measures that empower the EC and the Council to shape national fiscal governance in a way that they see will fit with the SGP. The timeframe of this research is limited to the end of the Juncker Commission (November 2019), but now the coronavirus pandemic is leading to a considerable shake-up of coordination mechanisms, precipitated notably by the triggering of a 'general escape clause' suspending corrective measures associated with fiscal governance (European Parliament, 2020). At the time of writing this book, it is still too early to tell how EU economic governance will unfold in the aftermath of the pandemic.

Going back to pre-pandemic era, one of the preventive tools that were introduced during the post-2008 fiscal reform is the European Semester. The European Semester is a cyclical policy coordination tool that assesses and coordinates the fiscal governance and sustainability of member states. It starts in October: before the submission of member states' budgets to national parliaments, member states submit their draft national budget to the EC. At that stage, the EC can ask member states to redraft their budget if it considers that it is incompatible with the SGP. In November, the EC publishes the EU yearly budgetary priorities (which includes the 'Annual growth survey'), the direction of which is already set out in the 7-year MFF. At this stage, the EC also publishes a report that flags up potential 'macroeconomic imbalances' that may result from member states' national budget plans, singling out those member states that will require 'in-depth review'. In March, the Council adopts the EU economic priorities based on the EC's reports. After that, in April, member states need to submit their fiscal plans and national reform programmes for the EC to review. National reform programmes are aimed at incorporating EU 2020 priorities at member state level and setting out a plan to reach EU targets, such as reducing unemployment, for example. Some of these targets were agreed in a soft governance setting and are now incorporated in the EU Semester process, which is why the Semester is seen as the link between soft EU 'social' governance and hard EU economic governance, subordinating the former to the latter (Greer et al., 2014).

Based on the scrutiny of the national fiscal plans and reform programmes, the EC elaborates 'country-specific recommendations'

(CSR), all with the view to ensuring member states align with the SGP. The CSR are then endorsed by the Council, discussed and adopted by the DG responsible for economic and financial affairs (DG ECFIN). While the Semester represents the 'preventive' arm of the fiscal compact, it does not preclude the possibility of sanctions for non-compliance (Delors et al., 2011; Köhler-Töglhofer, 2011; Savage & Howarth, 2017; Verdun & Zeitlin, 2017). Out of all the fiscal governance reforms and mechanisms to ensure compliance with the SGP, the Semester has been said to represent the 'softest' of tools. However, EU fiscal coordination should be considered in the category of hard governance because it is binding, and sanctions are applied in case of non-compliance. Greer has compared these tools to the structural adjustment programmes imposed on developing countries in the 1980s and 1990s (Greer, 2014b). The Semester might seem a softer tool at first sight, but because of its interlinkage with the other coordinating mechanisms, the degree to which the Semester represents merely a voluntary nudging tool is highly contentious.

'Soft' Governance

Soft governance refers to areas of governance in which the EU generally has only supportive (and shared) competencies and uses non-binding, voluntary means to promote integration. Those governing means have been referred to as 'new modes of governance' (NMG). Broadly speaking, hard governance is more widespread in economic areas of governance, and soft governance is more widespread in social areas of governance, which again is a consequence and cause of the maintenance of constitutional asymmetry. As such, the EU does not only regulate using hard law and binding coordination tools. Soft governance can be seen as the result of the drive to seek convergence between member states, but in places where the EU does not have clear treaty bases (see, for example, Radaelli, 2003; Schäfer, 2004). In those cases, promoting convergence can happen through coordinated learning, for example, through common research and innovation agenda, and through the tools of NMG.

After the Maastricht Treaty in 1992 and the creation of the EMU, the EU's governance areas were considerably extended to economic and social issues, including public health. However, the latter could not be done by applying the same 'supranational legislative' Community methods that had existed previously (notably for the Single Market), because the Treaty basis was too weak, and member states re-emphasised the importance of subsidiarity (Bruno et al., 2006). The early 1990s thus represented a time of further EU integration under the context of growing EU scepticism, including towards the single currency project, CAP reforms and the extension of EU competences to social areas (Bache et al., 2015). This 'legitimacy crisis' led the EU to creatively come up with other tools and modes of governance that would allow the EU project to be perceived as more democratically legitimate. This context is associated with the development of the NMG (Borrás & Jacobsson, 2004). NMG are soft, non-binding and more concerned with coordinating, steering and producing subjects than with dominating and coercing subjects. In attempting to promote a 'participatory' kind of governance, deemed more legitimate, these NMG also tend to bring every sector of society together, blurring the lines between the governing and the governed (Kohler-Koch & Rittberger, 2006). Generally speaking, NMG rely on voluntary cooperation and dialogue between stakeholders from all different sectors, including the public, private and voluntary sectors. The idea is to 'get everyone involved' to work towards common goals (commonly accepted by all, such as economic growth promotion, competition, but also social goals like good health or reduced inequalities) and to learn from each other and develop 'best practices'. Governing structures facilitate cooperation by offering a platform for dialogue and coordination (Eberlein & Kerwer, 2004). A key underlying assumption of NMG is that collaboration will lead to more efficient and more legitimate outcomes. There is also an anticipated peer pressure effect which would incentivise industry to commit to socially responsible behaviour. This rationale was pushed in particular by technocratic EU bodies like the EC, as opposed to the EP (which, in line with the institution's interest, takes a view on democratic legitimacy as strengthened through more power for elected representatives) (Smismans, 2003). In the case of the EU, the soft governance turn can be understood in relation to the commitments to increased participation and perhaps as a result of 'democratic experimentation'. The process of designing and using NMG further gained strength with the Lisbon Treaty (Diedrichs et al., 2011).

One of the most European 'democratic experiments' illustrating NMG is the OMC. The OMC is a tool of the Lisbon strategy. It is a form of soft law-making framework in which member states' representatives exchange best practices, set benchmarks and develop measurement indicators to tackle social issues which fall under member states' competence. The idea is that member states can learn from each other, learn from their differences and similarities and work together (Sabel & Zeitlin, 2008). The member states are expected to evaluate each other and learn from each other. The process is supervised by the EC, which does not directly intervene, and the outcomes are not legally binding (even though now they can be directly related to the EU fiscal governance, as suggested above). There is an OMC-*like* platform for member states' representatives to discuss public health promotion and NCD prevention: the HLG. It is not an OMC per se; however, the concept presents some similarity with OMCs insofar as member states' representatives come together to discuss ideas and exchange knowledge and experiences about health promotion and NCD prevention around healthy diet and physical activity promotion in particular.

'Meta-Regulatory' Governance

Meta-regulatory governance transcends the soft/hard divide and relates to 'the governance of governance'. Meta-regulatory governance relates to guidelines and processes about regulatory and decision-making processes. As such, it shapes the overall vision of the EU at the highest level, perhaps in the most influential but also least tangible way. Two examples of meta-regulatory elements—although very different in nature—include the Better Regulation agenda and the EC's principle of collegiality.

The EC is divided into two main sections, the College of Commissioners, which represents the political leadership of the EC and is appointed for five years, and various DGs, each headed by one commissioner, and which are the technical, supportive bodies of the EC. Each DG deals with a particular policy area; however, they are supposed to work together and make decisions with one single voice. As such, the EC shares a collective responsibility for its actions and has an obligation to follow the political guidelines established by the EC president (European Commission, 2000, p. 2). Any major decision (such as initiating new legislation or revising existing legislation, for example) needs to be approved by a simple majority in the College (European Commission, 2014, p. 4). The Juncker Commission working method emphasised the need for the EC to work closely together and improve the coherence and efficiency of EC actions by calling for the EU to be *big on big things and small on small things*. Its priorities were the following:

> a new boost for jobs, growth and investment, notably by means of a EUR 300bn investment plan; a connected Digital Single Market; a resilient

> European Energy Union with a forward-looking climate change policy; a deeper and fairer Internal Market with a strengthened industrial base, including a Capital Markets Union and based on the principle that the same work at the same place should be remunerated in the same manner; a deeper and fairer Economic and Monetary Union in which social dialogue is given new importance; a reasonable and balanced free trade agreement with the United States; an area of justice and fundamental rights based on mutual trust; a new EU policy on migration; making the EU a stronger global actor; and bringing about a Union of democratic change. (European Commission, 2014, p. 2)

This need for coherence and clear direction is part of the reason why certain commissioners have a 'vice-president' role. This means that their portfolio has a coordination element that cuts across the various DGs (European Commission, 2017a). Under the Juncker Commission (2014–2019), the DG in charge of health and food safety was abbreviated DG SANTE and was headed by Lithuanian Commissioner Vytenis Andriukaitis. The First Vice-President was Dutch politician Frans Timmermans, who was in charge, among other things, of coordinating the implementation of the Better Regulation agenda across the EC (European Commission, 2019a). The collegiality principle is still very much emphasised under the new von der Leyen presidency; however, it must be stated that the priorities and political directions have changed, in comparison with the Junker Commission. Frans Timmermans, for example, is still First Vice-President; however, his responsibilities are now centred more around implementing the European Green Deal (European Commission, 2019b).

The EC then works as a united block, and every commissioner is equally responsible for any EC decision. This is what is meant by the concept of 'collegiality'. The collegial decision-making process is based on regular (weekly) meetings of the College, as well as meetings of the heads of cabinets to prepare the work. Beyond decision-making, the College also uses 'orientation debates', which are debates about meta-regulation and meant to set the framework within which proposals should be developed and which reflect the broad, strategic political guidelines of the EC. The President does not consider new proposals unless they have been recommended by at least one of the vice-presidents, 'on the basis of sound argument and a clear narrative that is coherent with the priority projects of the Political Guidelines' (European Commission, 2014, p. 5).

As part of the collegiality requirement of the EC, inter-service consultations are launched by the relevant commissioner and in agreement with a vice-president, on any major initiative or proposal, prior to the political decision-making process. The consultation process is likely to feature notably consideration of impact assessments (IA) (European Commission, 2009, 2014).

This brings us to the other example of meta-regulation, the Better Regulation agenda. Better Regulation is a regulatory process agenda aimed at becoming a deeply embedded *way of working*. It dates to the 1990s but has gained strength over the last two decades in particular. It is a strongly present theme in both the Lisbon agenda and the Europe 2020 agenda. Better Regulation is part of a broader governance make-over which aims to simplify regulations by repealing outdated ones, cutting red tape and diversifying governance tools, favouring especially the use of non-binding tools.

Better Regulation is a meta-regulation with the ambition to 'improve' and simplify the regulatory process (Radaelli, 2007). It presents both structural and discursive properties:

> Better Regulation is a type of meta-regulation because of its emphasis on standards and rules which, instead of governing specific sectors or economic actors, steer the process of rule formulation, adoption, enforcement, and evaluation. (Radaelli, 2007 p. 191)

It is based on the principle that the EU should focus its actions on areas where it has the greatest added value, and that its involvement should be as minimal as possible without compromising the policy objectives (European Commission, 2015b). It is also about ensuring that the EU rules are 'fit for purpose, modern, effective, proportionate, operational and as simple as possible' (European Commission, 2015c, p. 4), via fitness-for-purpose evaluation cycles. The Better Regulation agenda includes various tools, which reflect the agenda's rationale for regulatory processes: impact assessment (IA), stakeholder consultation and ex-post evaluations (European Commission, 2015b). The Better Regulation documents put an emphasis on evidence and suggest that more openness of the regulatory process will lead to better evidence-informed regulations, through stakeholder consultations and IA (European Commission, 2015c). These tools were already important in the EU regulatory processes before the

Better Regulation agenda gained traction; however, the Juncker Commission's aim was to mainstream this agenda deeply and across the board, 'embedding Better Regulation in the Commission's DNA' (European Commission, 2017b, p. 2). This meta-regulatory project is intended to extend beyond the EC and become adopted by the EP, the Council and member states more generally (European Commission, 2015b). The EC developed the Regulatory Fitness and Performance (REFIT) Programme as part of the agenda to ensure continuous assessment of the quality and adequacy of existing regulations. The idea of REFIT is to modernise and update existing EU laws and regulations by targeting unnecessary burden, quantitatively estimating the cost that could be saved by optimising the regulation and embedding the REFIT tool into the EU political landscape (European Commission, 2015c). In summary, the Better Regulation logic underpins and permeates all the EC's work. It is based on three pillars: IA, stakeholder consultation and regulatory evaluation cycles to identify unnecessary 'red tape' that can be cut (European Commission, 2017b). Better regulation covers the whole policy cycle—planning, adoption, design, implementation, application (including enforcement), evaluation and revision (European Commission, 2017c, p. 6).

3.3 Conclusion: Broadening the Scope of EU Health Studies

This chapter has introduced some essentials of EU studies literature needed to get a sense of the EU's involvement in health and how it has been studied so far. In the light of concepts like constitutional asymmetry, we can start to see why the EU is a particularly interesting context to look at HiAP's lack of radical transformative power. Rather than taking it as a 'neoliberalism versus HiAP' dichotomy and thinking of HiAP as either present or absent, the idea here is to seek to better understand how framings, discourses and structures that maintain a 'neoliberal status quo' are reproduced and look at *how that shapes the meaning of HiAP*.

The impact of other EU areas on health has often been studied using the concept of spill over. This refers to, among other things, how the Single Market governance impacts on pharmaceuticals and medical devices, on patients' and health professionals' mobility, and how these constrain the capacity to take decisions on health systems at home. Greer's third face of EU involvement in health (through fiscal governance) is often thought in terms of EU meddling in national health system budgets under the pretext of the SGP. Building on this logic but focusing on improving macrosocial health determinants as health promotion, I suggest broadening the scope of what is commonly included in EU health studies. The relationship between EU fiscal governance and health, for example, should not be limited to national health system budget reduction (even though this is an important aspect), but needs to be extended to the whole palette of austerity measures (Karanikolos et al., 2013; Stuckler et al., 2017). The same applies to the second face of EU health involvement: the impact of Single Market integration on health should not be thought of as limited to direct encroachment on healthcare-related goods and services, but more broadly, any manifestation of political rationality which exacerbates societal inequities that should be considered harmful to health, essentially echoing the need to emphasise and expose the relationship between neoliberal rationality and ill-health—including with respect to NCDs. As for Greer's first face, i.e. engagement in public health through public health policies, it is important to analyse the kinds of paradigms and frames about health that these tools normalise and institutionalise.

To study this, we need to start from a radically broad conceptualisation of health promotion. If macrosocial determinants of health are to be taken seriously, then we need to engage with the role of power and political ideology as matters pertaining to health promotion. A radically broad conceptualisation of health promotion, along with the idea that health is to be mainstreamed, means that a lot of ground will have to be covered. The second part of this chapter provided a map to categorise EU governance into three types: hard, soft and meta-regulatory governance. The question of how HiAP will be studied across those governance types is addressed in the next chapter.

References

Anderson, K. M. (2015). *Social policy in the European Union*. Palgrave Macmillan.

Azzopardi-Muscat, N., Clemens, T., Stoner, D., & Brand, H. (2015). EU Country Specific Recommendations for health systems in the European Semester process: Trends, discourse and predictors. *Health Policy, 119*(3), 375–383.

Bache, I., Bulmer, S., George, S., & Parker, O. (2015). *Politics in the European Union* (4th ed.). Oxford University Press.

Bache, I., & Flinders, M. (Eds.). (2004). *Multi-level governance*. Oxford University Press.

Bailey, D. (2017). Obstacles to 'Social Europe.' In P. Kennett & N. Lendvai-Bainton (Eds.), *Handbook of European social policy* (pp. 108–125). Edward Elgar.

Baumberg, B., & Anderson, P. (2008). Health, alcohol and EU Law: Understanding the impact of European Single Market Law on alcohol policy. *European Journal of Public Health, 18*(4), 392–398.

Borrás, S., & Jacobsson, K. (2004). The open method of co-ordination and new governance patterns in the EU. *Journal of European Public Policy, 11*(2), 185–208.

Brooks, E. (2012). Crossing borders: A critical review of the role of the European Court of justice in EU health policy. *Health Policy, 105*, 33–37.

Bruno, I., Jacquot, S., & Mandin, L. (2006). Europeanization through its instrumentation: Benchmarking, mainstreaming and the open method of co-ordination...toolbox or Pandora's box? *Journal of European Public Policy, 13*(4), 519–536.

Buch-Hansen, H., & Wigger, A. (2010). Revisiting 50 years of market-making: The neoliberal transformation of European competition policy. *Review of International Political Economy, 17*(1), 20–44.

Cini, M. (2009). Intergovernmentalism. In M. Cini & N. Pérez-Solórzano Borragán (Eds.), *European Union Politics* (3rd ed., pp. 86–103). Oxford University Press.

Clemens, T., Sørensen, K., Rosenkotter, N., Michelsen, K., & Brand, H. (2017). The Directorate-General for Health and Consumers 1999–2014: An assessment of its functional capacities. *Health Policy, 121*(6), 594–603.

De Ruijter, A. (2019). *EU Health Law & Policy: The expansion of EU power in public health and health care*. Oxford University Press.

Delors, J., Fernandes, S., & Mermet, E. (2011, February). *The European Semester: Only a first step* [Policy Brief]. Notre Europe: Penser l'unité européenne No. 22.

Diedrichs, U., Reiners, W., & Wessels, W. (2011). New modes of governance policy development and the hidden steps of EU integration. In A. Heritier & M. Rhodes (Eds.), *New modes of governance in Europe* (pp. 19–47). Palgrave Macmillan.

Eberlein, B., & Kerwer, D. (2004). New governance in the European Union: A theoretical perspective. *Journal of Common Market Studies, 42*(1), 121–142.

EUR-Lex. (2010, August 5). Institutional balance of the European Union. *Official Journal of the European Union*. C 212 E/82. https://eur-lex.europa.eu/LexUriServ/LexUriServ.do?uri=OJ:C:2010:212E:0082:0093:EN:PDF. Accessed 4 May 2020.

European Commission. (2000). *Rules of procedure of the Commission* [C(2000) 3614]. https://op.europa.eu/en/publication-detail/-/publication/b1d6ec26-4815-4840-a903-329d42b1ab99. Accessed 12 November 2019.

European Commission. (2009, June 10). *Revised guide to interservice consultation and new instant statistics module in CIS-Net* [Note to Directors-General and Heads of Services]. https://ec.europa.eu/transparency/regdoc/rep/2/2009/EN/2-2009-780-EN-1-1.Pdf. Accessed 12 November 2019.

European Commission. (2014). *The working methods of the European Commission 2014–2019* [Communication from the President to the Commission]. https://ec.europa.eu/info/sites/info/files/the_working_methods_of_the_european_commission_2014-2019_november2014_en.pdf. Accessed 12 November 2019.

European Commission. (2015a). *Why we need a Digital Single Market*. https://ec.europa.eu/commission/sites/beta-political/files/dsm-factsheet_en.pdf. Accessed 12 November 2019.

European Commission. (2015b, May 19). *Proposal for an Interinstitutional Agreement on Better Regulation* [Communication from the Commission to the European Parliament and the Council]. Strasbourg. https://eur-lex.europa.eu/resource.html?uri=cellar:61fec455-fecb-11e4-a4c8-01aa75ed71a1.0001.02/DOC_1&format=PDF. Accessed 12 November 2019.

European Commission. (2015c, May 19). *Better regulation for better results – An EU agenda* [Communication from the Commission to the European Parliament, the European Economic and Social Committee and the Committee of the Regions] Strasbourg. https://eur-lex.europa.eu/legal-content/EN/TXT/PDF/?uri=CELEX:52015DC0215&from=EN. Accessed 12 November 2019.

European Commission. (2017a). *Governance in the European Commission* [Communication to the Commission from President Juncker and Vice-President Timmermans]. https://ec.europa.eu/info/sites/info/files/c_2017_6915_final_en.pdf. Accessed 12 November 2019.

European Commission. (2017b, October 24). *Completing the better regulation agenda* [Press Release]. PDF download available from: https://ec.europa.eu/commission/presscorner/detail/en/IP_17_4004. Accessed 12 November 2019.

European Commission. (2017c). *Better regulation 'toolbox'*. https://ec.europa.eu/info/sites/info/files/better-regulation-toolbox_2.pdf. Accessed 12 November 2019.

European Commission. (2019a). Decision of the President of the European Commission on the organisation of responsibilities of the Members of the Commission [Consolidated version]. https://ec.europa.eu/info/sites/info/files/decision-president-organisation-responsibilities-members-commission.pdf. Accessed 12 November 2019.

European Commission. (2019b, December 1). President von der Leyen's mission letter to Frans Timmermans. Brussels. https://ec.europa.eu/commission/commissioners/sites/comm-cwt2019/files/commissioner_mission_letters/mission-letter-frans-timmermans-2019_en.pdf. Accessed 15 May 2020.

European Parliament. (2018). 25 years of EU Single Market: Key achievements. http://www.europarl.europa.eu/resources/library/media/20180116RES91806/20180116RES91806.pdf. Accessed 12 November 2019.

European Parliament. (2020, March 27). *The 'general escape clause' within the Stability and Growth Pact: Fiscal flexibility for severe economic shocks*. https://www.europarl.europa.eu/thinktank/en/document.html. Accessed 7 March 2021.

European Union. (2003, February 8). Directive 2002/98/EC of the European Parliament and of the Council setting standards of quality and safety for the collection, testing, processing, storage, and distribution of human blood and blood components and amending Directive 2001/83/EC. *Official Journal of the European Union*. https://www.ema.europa.eu/en/documents/regulatory-procedural-guideline/directive-2002/98/ec-european-parliament-council-27-january-2003-setting-standards-quality-safety-collection-testing_en.pdf. Accessed 12 November 2019.

European Union. (2004a, July 12). Commission Recommendation on the transposition into national law of Directives affecting the internal market. *Official Journal of the European Union*. https://eur-lex.europa.eu/legal-content/EN/TXT/?uri=CELEX%3A32005H0309. Accessed 12 November 2019.

European Union. (2004b, April 7). Directive 2004/23/EC of the European Parliament and of the Council on setting standards of quality and safety for the donation, procurement, testing, processing, preservation, storage and distribution of human tissues and cells. *Official Journal of the European Union*. https://eur-lex.europa.eu/LexUriServ/LexUriServ.do?uri=OJ:L:2004:102:0048:0058:en:PDF. Accessed 12 November 2019.

European Union. (2011, March 9). Directive 2011/24/EU of the European Parliament and of the Council on the application of patient's rights in cross-border healthcare. *Official Journal of the European Union*. https://eur-lex.europa.eu/legal-content/EN/TXT/PDF/?uri=CELEX:32011L0024&from=EN. Accessed 12 November 2019.

European Union. (2016). *Division of competences within the European Union. Summaries of EU Legislation*. https://eur-lex.europa.eu/legal-content/EN/TXT/?uri=LEGISSUM%3Aai0020. Accessed 12 November 2019.

Fahy, N. (2012). Who is shaping the future of European health systems? *British Medical Journal, 344*(e1712). https://doi.org/10.1136/bmj.e1712

Ferrera, M. (2017). Mission impossible? Reconciling economic and social Europe after the euro crisis and Brexit. The Stein Rokkan Lecture 2016. *European Journal of Political Research, 56*, 3–22.

Flear, M. (2015). *Governing public health: EU law, regulation and biopolitics*. Hart Publishing.

Garde, A. (2010). *EU law and obesity prevention*. Alphen aan den Rijn: Kluwer Law International.

Geyer, R., & Lightfoot, S. (2010). The strengths and limits of new forms of EU Governance: The case of mainstreaming and impact assessment in EU Public Health and sustainable development policy. *European Integration, 32*(4), 339–356.

Gill, S. (1998). European Governance and new constitutionalism: Economic and Monetary Union and alternatives to disciplinary neoliberalism in Europe. *New Political Economy, 3*(1), 5–26.

Greer, S. L. (2006). Uninvited Europeanization: Neofunctionalism and the EU in health policy. *Journal of European Public Policy, 13*(1), 134–152.

Greer, S. L. (2009). *The politics of European Union health policies*. Open University Press.

Greer, S. L. (2014a). Three faces of European Union Health Policy: Policy, markets, and austerity. *Policy and Society, 33*(1), 13–24.

Greer, S. L. (2014b). Structural adjustment comes to Europe: Lessons for the Eurozone from the Conditionality Debates. *Global Social Policy, 14*(1), 51–71.

Greer, S. L., Fahy, N., Heather, A. E., Wismar, M., Jarman, H., Palm, W., Elliott, H. A., & Wismar, M. (2014). *Everything you always wanted to know about European Union health policies but were too afraid to ask*. The European Observatory on Health Systems and Policies. Tetragon.

Greer, S. L., & Löblová, O. (2016). European integration in the era of permissive dissensus: Neofunctionalism and agenda-setting in European health technology assessment and communicable disease control. *Comparative European Politics, 15*(3), 394–413.

Guy, M., & Sauter, W. (2017). The history and scope of EU health law and policy. In T. Hervey, C. Young, & L. Bishop (Eds.), *Research handbook on EU Health Law and Policy* (pp. 17–35). Edward Elgar.

Haas, E. B. (1958). *The uniting of Europe: Political, Social, and Economic Forces 1950–1957*. University of Notre Dame Press.

Hall, D. (2002). EU competition policies and public services. *Transfer: European Review of Labour and Research, 8*(2), 198–2013.

Héritier, A. (2001). Market integration and social cohesion: The politics of public services in European regulation. *Journal of European Public Policy, 8*(5), 825–852.

Jacquot, S. (2010). The paradox of gender mainstreaming: Unanticipated effects of new modes of governance in the gender equality domain. *West European Politics, 33*(1), 118–135.

Jensen, C. S. (2009). Neo-functionalism. In M. Cini & N. Pérez-Solórzano Borragán (Eds.), *European Union politics* (3rd ed., pp. 71–85). Oxford University Press.

Karanikolos, M., Mladovsky, P., Cylus, J., Thomson, S., Basu, S., Stuckler, D., Mackenbach, J. P., McKee, M. (2013). Financial crisis, austerity, and health in Europe. *The Lancet, 381*(9874), 1323–1331.

Kohler-Koch, B., & Rittberger, B. (2006). Review article: The 'Governance Turn' in EU Studies. *Journal of Common Market Studies, 44*, 27–49.

Köhler-Töglhofer, W. (2011). Macro coordination under the European Semester. *Monetary Policy and the Economy* [Österreichische Nationalbank], issue 4, 59–73.

Lamping, W. (2005). European integration and health policy: A peculiar relationship. In M. Steffen (Ed.), *Health governance in Europe: Issues, challenges and theories* (pp. 18–48). Routledge.

Lamping, W., & Steffen, M. (2009). European Union and Health Policy: The "Chaordic" dynamics of integration. *Social Science Quarterly, 90*(5), 1361–1379.

Liebfried, S. (2010). Social policy: Left to the judges and the markets? In H. Wallace, M. A. Pollack, & A. Young (Eds.), *Policy-making in the European Union* (6th ed., pp. 253–282). Oxford University Press.

Majone, G. (1993). The European Community between social policy and social regulation. *Journal of Common Market Studies, 31*(2), 153–170.

Majone, G. (2014). From regulatory state to a democratic default. *Journal of Common Market Studies, 52*(6), 1216–1223.

Melkas, T. (2013). Health in All Policies as a priority in Finnish health policy: A case study on national health policy development. *Scandinavian Journal of Public Health, 41*(Suppl. 11), 3–28.

Moravcsik, A. (1998). *The choice for Europe: Social purpose & state power from Messina to Maastricht*. Routledge.

Mossialos, E., Permanand, G., Baeten, R., & Hervey, T. (2010). Health systems governance in Europe: The role of European Union Law and Policy. In E. Mossialos, G. Permanand, R. Baeten, & T. Hervey (Eds.), *Health systems governance in Europe: The role of European Union Law and Policy* (pp. 1–83). Cambridge University Press.

Niemann, A., & Ioannou, D. (2015). European economic integration in times of crisis: A case of neofunctionalism? *Journal of European Public Policy, 22*(2), 196–218.

Parker, O. (2018). A genealogy of EU discourses and practices of deliberative governance: Beyond states and markets? *Public Administration, 97*, 741–753.

Parker, O., & Pye, R. (2018). Mobilising social rights in EU economic governance: A pragmatic challenge to neoliberal Europe. *Comparative European Politics, 16*, 805–824.

Pollack, M. (2001). International relations theory and European Integration. *Journal of Common Market Studies, 39*(2), 221–244.

Radaelli, C. (2003, March). *The open method of coordination: A new governance architecture for the European Union?* Swedish Institute for European Policy Studies [Rapport no. 1].

Radaelli, C. (2007). Whither better regulation for the Lisbon agenda? *Journal of European Public Policy, 14*(2), 190–207.

Rosamond, B. (2002). Imagining the European Economy: 'Competitiveness' and the social construction of 'Europe' as an economic space. *New Political Economy, 7*(2), 157–177.

Rosamond, B. (2009). New theories of European integration. In M. Cini & N. Pérez-Solórzano Borragán (Eds.), *European Union politics* (3rd ed., pp. 104–122). Oxford University Press.

Sabel, C. F., & Zeitlin, J. (2008). Learning from difference: The new architecture of experimentalist governance in the EU. *European Law Journal, 14*(3), 271–327.

Savage, J. D., & Howarth, D. (2017). Enforcing the European semester: The politics of asymmetric information in the excessive deficit and macroeconomic imbalance procedure. *Journal of European Public Policy, 25*(2), 212–230.

Schäfer, A. (2004). Beyond the community method: Why the open method of coordination was introduced to EU policy-making. *European Integration Online Papers (EIoP), 8*(13).

Scharpf, F. (1997, November). *Balancing positive and negative integration: The regulatory options for Europe* (MPIfG Working Paper 97/8). http://www.mpifg.de/pu/workpap/wp97-8/wp97-8.html. Accessed 11 November 2019.

Scharpf, F. (1998). Negative and positive Integration in the Political Economy of European Welfare States. In M. Rhodes & Y. Meny (Eds.), *The future of European welfare: A new social contract?* (pp. 155–177). Palgrave.

Scharpf, F. (2002). The European social model: Coping with the challenges of diversity. *Journal of Common Market Studies, 40*(4), 645–670.

Scharpf, F. (2006). The joint-decision trap revisited. *Journal of Common Market Studies, 44*(4), 845–864.

Siles-Brügge, G. (2013). The power of economic ideas: A constructivist political economy of EU Trade Policy. *Journal of Contemporary European Research, 9*(4), 597–617.

Sindbjerg Martinsen, D. (2017). Governing EU Health Law and Policy: On Governance and Legislative Politics. In T. Hervey, C. Young, & L. Bishop (Eds.), *Research Handbook on EU Health Law and Policy* (pp. 36–59). Edward Elgar.

Smismans, S. (2003). European civil society: Shaped by discourses and institutional interests. *European Law Journal, 9*(4), 473–495.

Staab, A. (2013). *The European Union explained*. Indiana University Press.

Steffen, M., Lamping, W., & Lehto, J. (2005). The Europeanization of health policies. In M. Steffen (Ed.), *Health governance in Europe: Issues, challenges and theories* (pp. 1–17). Routledge.

Stuckler, D., Reeves, A., Loopstra, R., Karanikolos, M., & McKee, M. (2017). Austerity and health: The impact in the UK and Europe. *European Journal of Public Health, 27*(Suppl. 4), 18–21.

Van Apeldoorn, B., Drahokoupil, J., & Horn, L. (Eds.). (2009). *Contradictions and limits of neoliberal European governance: From Lisbon to Lisbon*. Palgrave.

Van Apeldoorn, B., & Horn, L. (2018, May). *Critical political economy* (Working Paper, KFG The Transformative Power of Europe. No. 87).

Van Gerven, M., & Ossewaarde, M. (2018). Beyond the neoliberal paradigm? Images of Social Europe in open method of coordination employment peer reviews. *Social Policy and Administration, 52*, 1354–1366.

Verdun, A., & Zeitlin, J. (2017). Introduction: The European Semester as a new architecture of EU socioeconomic governance in theory and practice. *Journal of European Public Policy, 25*(2), 137–148.

Walters, W., & Haahr, J. H. (2005). *Governing Europe: Discourse, governmentality and European integration*. Routledge.

CHAPTER 4

How Can We Research 'Health in All Policies' in the EU?

This chapter sets out a discursive institutionalist (DI) framework (see Schmidt, 2008, 2015) to look at dynamics of institutional continuity and change in relation to HiAP in the EU. DI thinks of institutions as social and discursive constructs that shape and are shaped by the people that make up those institutions. On the one hand, this framework locates structural continuity in both 'formal' institutional architecture and ideational power dynamics that maintain established belief systems (notably dominant ways of understanding health and the knowledge/policy relationship). On the other hand, it locates the space for agential change (though not necessarily radical change) in the discursive characteristics of HiAP: how has HiAP been articulated and how has it evolved since? What explains the relative success of HiAP reaching the EU in the first place? If radical change is unlikely, could HiAP still foster some kind of slow, gradual change? Looking at both structural and agential power dynamics prevents overly deterministic depictions of institutions, without over-estimating the scope for change. In this chapter, I argue that analysing structural (ideational and institutional) constraints, as well as HiAP itself, enables us to critically evaluate its potential to induce change.

C. Godziewski, *The Politics of Health Promotion*, Palgrave Studies in Science, Knowledge and Policy, https://doi.org/10.1007/978-3-030-97870-9_4

4.1 Institutional Change and Continuity

Unpacking the relative failure of HiAP at EU level, while also exploring its potential, requires looking at various kinds of power dynamics. It requires analysing institutional change and continuity, and the potential for ideas to bring about such change. Varieties of institutionalist theories have been concerned with these questions, and they have sought to define institutions and explain how they 'work', and how and why they evolve in certain ways.

Since the 1990s in particular, 'new institutionalist' theories started developing and becoming increasingly popular in studying the institutional functioning of the EU, with a focus on the concept of governance. The term 'new institutionalism' commonly refers to three variants of institutionalism: rational choice institutionalism, historical institutionalism and sociological institutionalism. Arguably, these institutionalisms all tend to conceptualise institutions as relatively rigid, inert and constraining structures. This means that these approaches tend to see institutional continuity as the norm, and changes as resulting from exogenous shocks. More recently, and moving on from these forms of new institutionalisms, researchers concerned with studying institutional change and continuity started directing their attention to the power of ideas and discourse. Elements of different institutionalisms inform each other, and the boundaries between different variants can be fluid. But overall, the growing concern with ideas and discourse stems from a felt need to 'endogenize institutional change' (Schmidt, 2010a, p. 2). That is, the need to find a better way to understand institutional change as more than the result of external shocks, recognise the space for incremental change produced from within and consider the role of ideas and discourses more seriously. This can be seen as a response to the (arguably) overly deterministic nature of new institutionalisms (Gorges, 2001; Schmidt, 2010a). This evolution, then, represents a constructivist turn of institutionalism, rejecting both the idea that agents existing within institutions are rational actors with predictable, rational interests and the idea that institutional evolution is necessarily historically or culturally pre-determined (Blyth, 2002; Hay, 2010).

Discursive institutionalism (DI) is one prominent example of constructivist theoretical approaches which evaluate the role of ideas, discourse and institutions to understand institutional change and continuity. Vivien Schmidt defines DI as 'an umbrella concept for approaches that concern themselves with the substantive content of ideas and the interactive processes of discourse in institutional context' (Schmidt, 2015, p. 1). It is a label that can be attributed to any research concerned with the study of the interplay between ideas and discourses within an institutional context (Schmidt, 2017). The most relevant elements of DI are:

1. A conceptualisation of institutions as socially and discursively constructed, as simultaneously constraining agents in what they can think and do and produced/shaped by these agents. Institutions are not seen as neutral, objectively pre-existing entities, but they are the product of normatively driven social construction. They are both constraining structures that shape what can be done and how actors can behave within them, as well as enabling constructs, which come about through a combination of underlying rationalities which shape what is thinkable, as well as individual actors' agency within them. This points to the non-inevitability of the way in which institutions are at one moment in time, acknowledging the scope for change and evolution, while at the same time recognising the obstacles to change.
2. A focus on ideational power. Ideational power is defined in DI as 'the capacity of actors (whether individual or collective) to influence other actors' normative and cognitive beliefs through the use of ideational elements' (Carstensen & Schmidt, 2016, p. 321). This can take place in different ways, such as with power *though* ideas, power *over* ideas and power *in* ideas. Ideational power can thus mean various things simultaneously: power *through* ideas refers to mechanisms like persuasion, and the ability to challenge others to think outside their 'institutional box'. Power *over* ideas represents the power to attribute and define the meaning of ideas. Power *in* ideas represents the authority that certain ideas have, whereas others become dismissed out of hand and are not even discussed. Depoliticisation, for example, is one form of power *in* ideas (Carstensen & Schmidt, 2016).
3. The need to take into account three overlapping and co-constitutive elements: the *institutional context*, *background ideational abilities* which constrain and shape the way in which the world is predominantly made sense of within the institution, and *foreground discursive abilities* of agents within institutions who have the capacity to articulate a discourse critical (or not) of their own institutions (Schmidt,

Table 4.1 Applying the theoretical framework in practice: summative table

	Chapter 5	*Chapter 6*	*Chapter 7*
DI element	Institutional context	Background ideational structures	Foreground discursive abilities
Object of study in relation to HiAP	EU institutional architecture	Dominant paradigms and frames around health and scientific evidence	Active shaping and redefining of HiAP
Form of power	Institutional power	Power *in* ideas	Power *through* and *over* ideas
Emphasis	Structure *(although evolving, not pre-determined)*	Structure *(although evolving, not pre-determined)*	Agency *(although not entirely independent of structure)*

2010a, 2010b, 2015). Importantly, these three elements are overlapping and co-constituted. Background ideational abilities, in this book, are seen as pertaining more to structure than to agency and will therefore be referred to as 'background ideational structures'.[1]

The remaining chapters will be structured along those three elements (see Table 4.1). The chapter on institutional context will focus on how institutional power dynamics, such as constitutional asymmetry, affect HiAP. The chapter on background ideational structures will focus on power *in* ideas and look at how certain cognitive frames and paradigms around health and evidence narrow the scope of HiAP. The chapter on foreground discursive abilities will focus on power *through* and *over* ideas and unpack the discursive struggles around the meaning and definition of HiAP itself. This multitude of forms of power allows for a nuanced

[1] Rather than taking as a starting point the dynamic discursive processes and then analysing their contents, it takes the ideas underpinning discourses as the starting point and then analyses how these are reproduced as well as challenged. Conceptually, this means that, instead of putting the agent in the middle of the analysis and considering how structure acts upon it, this book puts the structure (institutional and ideational) in the centre, and then considers how the agent can nevertheless challenge and change it. Therefore, this book conceptualises background ideas as structures rather than as abilities. Ingrained background ideational structures may indeed have stemmed from particular agents successfully articulating ideas in a way that they ended up becoming unquestioned and fading into the background.

analysis of structure and agency, highlighting the balance between continuity pull and the push for change. Using this approach to look at HiAP in the EU is particularly interesting, because it allows us to explore how HiAP became a concept used in the EU, despite the prevailing institutional neoliberal bias, how it has both successfully made its way to the EU and failed to spark fundamental change. Using DI offers the possibility for a nuanced analysis of the interactions between prevailing (neoliberal) ideational frames (e.g. frames of health and NCDs, as well as frames of what constitutes evidence), institutional structures that reflect constitutional asymmetry and the space for contestation in the very idea of HiAP, as well as in its actively driven evolution.

4.2 The Pull Towards Continuity: Prevailing Ideas and Institutions

Institutional Context

Before delving in the discursive and ideational dynamics that affect how HiAP is understood and what it can do, it makes sense to start with looking at the obvious starting point: the 'formal' institutional scene. What kind of institutional context did HiAP enter when it was introduced at EU level in 2006? As we have already seen in the previous chapter, EU institutions present an ingrained asymmetry towards market integration. With that in mind, it is useful to start with an overview of the (limited) space for HiAP in the EU 'formal' institutions architecture. There is a vast literature explaining the constitutionally asymmetrical power dynamics driving EU integration. Some have already looked at the implications of these asymmetries on the EU's involvement in health (especially healthcare) policy and law. Others have used the notion of constitutional asymmetry to explore the neoliberal biases of EU integration. However, these insights have not yet been explored as much in relation to health promotion, the macrosocial determinants of health and the health mainstreaming agenda.

Although the point of DI is to look *beyond* 'traditional' conceptualisations of institutional structures, the insights from the 'older' new institutionalisms contribute to the overall analysis: what path dependencies and historical developments shape the institutional context, what norms have become established in that space over time, and how institutional structures are skewed in ways that favour certain interests over others.

These aspects are contextual rather than central to DI, because they are less concerned with ideas per se. However, it is important to take those structures as a starting point, especially given that DI considers institutional context and ideational/discursive dynamics as co-constitutive. Treaties matter, and institutions do not exist as purely cognitive structures, without context. HiAP within the institutional context will be the object of a dedicated chapter. It will draw on the concept of constitutional asymmetry to analyse the space for HiAP in selected examples of EU soft, hard and meta-regulatory governance.

Background Ideational Structures

Background ideas, in DI, are ingrained representations of the world, commonly accepted, taken-for-granted 'truths'. They are not explicitly articulated but tend to be taken as 'common knowledge', 'obvious', simply the logical way to make sense of a particular phenomenon. Background ideas tend to develop a life of their own, even shaping reality by providing a lens through which phenomena are made sense of. These background ideas infuse how people think about themselves and the world, how policymakers make sense of social phenomena, and how the policies aimed to solve them are designed. The ideational background is constructed through established 'power *in* ideas', which, as Carstensen and Schmidt (2016) puts it, concerns:

> [...] the ways that agents seek to depoliticise ideas to the degree where they recede into the background, meaning that they become so accepted that their very existence may be forgotten, even as they may come to structure people's thoughts about the economy, polity and society. (p. 329)

Ascertaining whether background ideas are the result of agency or structure is not the point here. That depends on whether agents are considered active 'discourse users' or whether they are considered almost 'a product of discourse' (Bacchi, 2005). It is reasonable to assume that it might be an unknowable mix of both. But given that a certain set of background ideas is, at a moment in time, successfully ingrained, they will be thought of herein more in terms of structure (not pre-determined and fixed, but slowly evolving structure), regardless of the extent to which they initially originated from agency. Typically, an idea like neoliberalism represents a worldview-structuring, taken-for-granted idea that has become so accepted that it fades into the background while guiding what is thinkable and sayable (Schmidt, 2016). This kind of authority of ideas is described as being situated at a 'deeper level' than policy ideas or programmes, as being left unarticulated yet shaping the realm of possibilities of how to even think about reality, the realm of what is acceptable to think. However, even this kind of power is not pre-determined and immutable, even though changes here tend to occur very slowly. To theorise this power *in* ideas, especially in the context of neoliberalism, Carstensen and Schmidt (2016, pp. 330–331) draw on Foucault's governmentality (see also: Panizza & Miorelli, 2013). What this means is that, even though DI so far has tended to take a more agency-oriented approach and focus more on power *through* and *over* ideas, it does not neglect the ideational constraints composed of underlying, taken-for-granted worldviews. However (and this is in line with Foucauldian approaches as well), DI still emphasises that, however difficult and slow the change process may be, background ideational structures are not inevitably pre-determined and do evolve.

To look at relevant elements of background ideational landscape prevailing at EU level and which have an impact on how HiAP can operate, I use Rushton and Williams' (2012) 'Framework for Analysing Global Health Policymaking'. This framework sheds light on how global health policymaking is shaped discursively, through interaction between by frames, paradigms and power.

'Frames' refer to linguistic and cognitive devices at the most 'immediate level' of discursive construction of a problem (Rushton & Williams, 2012). Their presence implies that global health issues, or any kind of phenomena for that matter, do not exist objectively 'out there', but are constructed and made sense of discursively. Frames lie in the cognitive foreground of actors. 'Paradigms' refer to background cognitive devices that inform frames. They are situated in the background of frames (they 'frame the frames'). Examples of paradigms informing global health frames and policies mentioned include the economic paradigm, or the biomedical paradigm among others. Power, in this framework, relates to the agency of certain groups to shape the frames and shape the policies. However, all these dimensions: frames, paradigms and power, are underpinned by what they call an overarching 'deep core', which determines what is doable, sayable and thinkable in the very first place. The deep core, according to them, is neoliberalism.

> [...]the hegemony of the neoliberal orthodoxy results in a situation where all of the paradigms of global health exist and develop in a context defined by neoliberal ideas. (Rushton & Williams, 2012, p. 165)

The processes that relate deep core with paradigm and frames need to be traced and studied empirically. Chapter 6 will draw on this framework to investigate the background ideational structures dominating in EU health governance. This will allow to unpack manifestations of the 'deep core', manifestations of neoliberalism through paradigms and frames that undermine a normatively meaningful HiAP shift at EU level. The aim of that part of the book will be to look at the relationship between deep core neoliberalism, paradigms of health and of knowledge, and frames of NCDs and of evidence. As such, this chapter is particularly concerned with what Schmidt calls the power *in* ideas. How do obstacles to a normative HiAP manifest through existing background ideational structures that provide a frame within which to make sense of the world, including of HiAP? These background ideational power dynamics have implications for how much HiAP can do.

4.3 The Push for Change? Discourses, Redefinition and Recycling

On the one hand, DI zooms into how structures, both formal and ideational, maintain institutional continuity. As we will see, this provides a less than hospitable setting for HiAP to be meaningfully taken up. But by using DI, we also want to avoid overly deterministic depictions of EU institutions as monolithically and inevitably neoliberal. That is why looking at HiAP itself and the active, 'agential' discourses and definitions of this idea matters. Of course, the division between structure and agency is not as clear-cut, but nevertheless, for analytical purposes, it is useful to think in those terms at least to flesh out some of the power dynamics around HiAP in the EU.

Looking at HiAP as an active discourse allows us to investigate how HiAP is defined, and how its definition is negotiated, and why. Where are more radical HiAP discourses articulated, if at all? How do proponents of HiAP discursively react to the challenges the idea faces in the EU setting? The 'foreground discursive abilities' element of DI allows us to some of the endogenous (and incremental) change happening. They have been the focus of most DI scholars (see amongst others also: Boswell &

Hampshire, 2017; Herranz-Surrallés, 2012; Wahlström & Sundberg, 2018). This entails zooming in on the 'power *through* ideas' and 'power *over* ideas' angles of ideational power (as opposed to ideational structures which relates more to 'power *in* ideas').

But the term discourse is contentious and can mean quite different things depending on who is using it. For DI scholars who draw on deliberative democracy, discourse refers to a Habermasian idea of communicative action (Dryzek, 1990). In those cases, DI scholars are particularly interested in looking at the discrepancies between coordinative discourses, through which policymakers construct policies behind closed doors, and communicative discourses, which occur in the interactions between policymakers and the general public (both top-down and/or bottom-up), and where policies are discursively legitimated and/or contested. Discourse, in part, refers to the discursive process—the 'who said what to whom?' (Schmidt, 2008, p. 305). Focusing on the process angle will entail an exploration of power *through* ideas and coercive power. Power *over* ideas refers to 'the politics of attributing meaning to ideas' and refers to the content, more than the process, of discourse. The term discourse as used by Schmidt (2015) encompasses both the content and the process:

> the representation or embodiment of ideas – as in discourse analysis [...] but also the interactive process by and through which ideas are generated in the policy sphere by discursive policy communities and entrepreneurs [...] and communicated, deliberated, and/or contested in the political sphere by political leaders, social movements and the public [...]. (p. 171)

Both content and process are co-constitutive, and therefore power *over* and *through* ideas cannot be neatly separated. In Chapter 7, I will consider both together, as my main concern is with the malleability of the meaning of HiAP: power *through* ideas is the discursive effort to persuade others of the validity of one's idea, illustrated in the strategic adaptation of the meaning of ideas to persuade others to take it up in the first place. The introduction of HiAP into the EU space in 2006, represents an instance of power *through* ideas, where the Finnish team sought to convince the EU officials of the importance and validity of health mainstreaming as an idea. Power *over* ideas' is the active power struggle to define the meaning of HiAP, illustrated in the adaptation of the meaning of ideas to redefine them 'once taken up'. What happened to HiAP after its introduction, the power struggles to redefine and delimit its meaning, relates to power *over* ideas.

The purpose of Chapter 7, then, is to look at the various (contradictory) meanings of HiAP, where they take place, and by whom these various meanings are put forward. This will allow for a better insight into the space for (gradual, incremental) institutional (and ideational) change, without being overly optimistic and recognising the struggles for HiAP advocates to resist the risk of co-option. To do so, it will draw on Smith's (2013) categorisation of ideas. She categorises four types of ideas, including one type she calls 'chameleonic ideas'. This concept refers to ideas that are formulated vaguely enough to appeal to various audiences. In relation to public health research, these often refer to ideas that have been 'strategically packaged' to be perceived as acceptable in mainstream governance. Ultimately, identifying chameleonic qualities of ideas points to the fact that meanings of ideas are not fixed and can be challenged and changed. Furthermore, meanings of ideas are not only changeable, but various contradictory meanings of chameleonic ideas and concepts can co-exist. The last parts of the book will investigate how HiAP can become fitted to the dominant EU neoliberal rationality. At the same time, HiAP can also be a space for agency in which actors within an institution can articulate discourses critical of that institution. This is visible in the actively driven evolution and 'recycling' of HiAP into the 'economy of wellbeing' idea. Furthermore, HiAP is a very broad and normative concept. Consequently, various different ideas can share a same normative vision with HiAP, without necessarily being called 'HiAP'. That may be the case for more radical ideas like the 'degrowth' movement.

4.4 Conclusion: Taking into Account Multiple Kinds of Power

DI is concerned with how ideational power and discursive practices interact with institutional context to maintain or change it. In the case of this book, the main characteristics of the institutional context have been introduced in the previous Chapter 3, specifically the notion of 'constitutional asymmetry', and how it creates an ingrained neoliberal bias that favours economic integration over social integration. However, institutional context alone cannot explain either why HiAP made its way to the EU in the first place, nor does it explain what happens to this idea once it reached that space. In other words, looking at health in the EU purely from a constitutional asymmetry angle would provide an overly deterministic picture, which would invariably point towards the inevitable reproduction of neoliberalism. In quite a similarly deterministic way, some research drawing on governmentality to critically analyse neoliberal rationality also tends to end up seeing neoliberal governmentality everywhere and consistently, and seeing deep philosophical ideas as never changing (Schmidt, 2015). This becomes equally unhelpful, as pointed out by those sympathetic to the concept of governmentality, but keen to draw more attention to and put more weight on agency, and the non-inevitability of current domination of rationalities (Bell & Green, 2016; Cairns & Johnston, 2015). The problem with painting a totalising picture of neoliberal governmentality is that it would negate the whole point of looking at discourse and ideas. Put simply, if the discourse is omnipresent and always coherently neoliberal, then one might as well call it an institution.

In contrast, DI offers a useful framework to use to analyse HiAP at EU level. It allows for striking a balance between structure and agency when looking at the effects and promotion of ideas intended to foster institutional change. It combines a sophisticated conceptualisation of power which considers the interplay of ideational structures and institutions, but without neglecting the space for agency, the possibility for agents to also reflect critically upon the institution within which they act, and perhaps even their own normative assumptions.

The following chapters will focus on one of the three components of DI and its respectively most relevant form of power: Chapter 5 will deal with the institutional context and *institutional* power, Chapter 6 for background ideational structures and power *in* ideas, and Chapter 7 will look at foreground discursive abilities and power *over* and *through* ideas (Fig. 4.1).

It is important to bear in mind that the separation of the three elements (institutional context, background ideational structures and foreground discursive abilities) is created for analytical purposes. All three elements are better seen as co-constitutive. For example, the institutional context is constructed by both the reproduction of established background ideas and the discursive agency of sentient beings in that institution. Institutional context and background ideas are mutually reinforcing. Foreground discourses do not exist in a vacuum, and while they may well be critical of institutional continuity, they cannot be seen as entirely separate from background ideas, with the former potentially even coming to shape the latter in the long run.

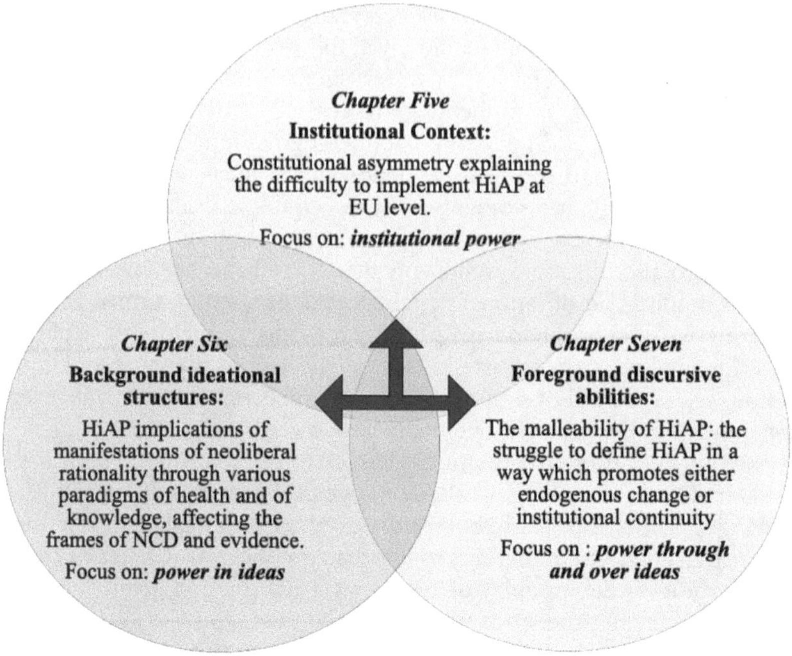

Fig. 4.1 Structure of the analysis

Ultimately, DI allows for a sophisticated analysis of institutional change and continuity, in a way that aims to avoid over-emphasising individual agency (i.e. to understand the structural constraints beyond simply institutional ones), but without falling into overly deterministic accounts of institutions. The relative emphases on these different aspects, according to Schmidt, are up to the researcher to position themselves towards, as she sees her framework as a broad umbrella framework capable of including different types of research.

References

Bacchi, C. (2005). Discourse, discourse everywhere: Subject "agency" in feminist discourse methodology. *Nordic Journal of Women's Studies, 13*(3), 198–209.

Bell, K., & Green, J. (2016). On the perils of invoking neoliberalism in public health critique. *Critical Public Health, 26*(3), 239–243.

Blyth, M. (2002). *Great transformations: Economic ideas and institutional change in the twentieth century*. Cambridge University Press.
Boswell, C., & Hampshire, J. (2017). Ideas and agency in immigration policy: A discursive institutionalist approach. *European Journal of Political Research, 56*, 133–150.
Cairns, K., & Johnston, J. (2015). Choosing health: Embodied neoliberalism, post-feminism, and the do-diet. *Theory and Society, 44*(2), 153–175.
Carstensen, M. B., & Schmidt, V. (2016). Power through, over and in Ideas: Conceptualizing ideational power in discursive institutionalism. *Journal of European Public Policy, 23*(3), 318–337.
Dryzek, J. S. (1990). *Discursive democracy: Politics, policy and political science*. Cambridge University Press.
Gorges, M. J. (2001). The new institutionalism and the study of the European Union: The case of the social dialogue. *West European Politics, 24*(4), 152–168.
Hay, C. (2010). Ideas and the construction of interests. In D. Beland & R. Cox (Eds.), *Ideas and politics in social science research* (pp. 65–82). Oxford University Press.
Herranz-Surrallés, A. (2012). Justifying enlargement in a multi-level polity: A discursive institutionalist analysis of the elites-public gap over European Union enlargement. *Journal of Common Market Studies, 50*(3), 385–402.
Panizza, F., & Miorelli, R. (2013). Taking discourse seriously: Discursive institutionalism and post-structuralist discourse theory. *Political Studies, 61*(2), 301–318.
Rushton, S., & Williams, O. D. (2012). Frames, paradigms and power: Global health policy-making under neoliberalism. *Global Society, 26*(2), 147–167.
Schmidt, V. (2008). Discursive institutionalism: The explanatory power of ideas and discourse. *The Annual Review of Political Science, 11*, 303–326.
Schmidt, V. (2010a). Taking ideas and discourse seriously: Explaining change through discursive institutionalism as the fourth 'new institutionalism.' *European Political Science Review, 2*(1), 1–25.
Schmidt, V. (2010). Reconciling ideas and institutions through discursive institutionalism. In D. Beland & R. Cox (Eds.), *Ideas and politics in social science research* (pp. 47–64). Oxford University Press.
Schmidt, V. (2015). Discursive institutionalism: Understanding policy in context. In F. Fischer, D. Torgerson, & A. Durnova (Eds.), *Handbook of critical policy studies* (pp. 171–189). Edward Elgar.
Schmidt, V. (2016). The roots of neo-liberal resilience: Explaining continuity and change in background ideas in Europe's political economy. *The British Journal of Politics and International Relations, 18*(2), 318–334.

Schmidt, V. (2017). Theorizing ideas and discourse in political science: Intersubjectivity, neo-institutionalism, and the power of ideas. *Critical Review, 29*(2), 248–263.
Smith, K. E. (2013). *Beyond evidence-based policy in public health: The interplay of ideas*. Palgrave Macmillan.
Wahlström, N., & Sundberg, D. (2018). Discursive institutionalism: Towards a framework for analysing the relation between policy and curriculum. *Journal of Education Policy, 33*(1), 163–183.

CHAPTER 5

Setting the Scene: Are EU Institutions 'HiAP-Friendly'?

In the previous chapter, I argued that structural constraints on HiAP are both institutional ('traditionally' understood) and ideational in nature. This chapter unpacks the former type of constraint. It draws on existing research on constitutional asymmetry to detail how the EU institutions are shaped in a way that leaves HiAP unable to reach the spaces in which macrosocial determinants of health are governed. Those spaces include most notably the regulation of the Single Market, economic and fiscal coordination, as well as the meta-regulatory processes that shape the policymaking and governance architecture. By contrast, the spaces explicitly dedicated to public health are institutionally much weaker. They are either kept separate from macrosocial determinants of health, or they become subordinated to the goals of other policy areas. Exploring a range of examples, this chapter shows how the EU institutional context is not favourable to HiAP. This observation, in and of itself, is neither novel, nor surprising. However, given its focus on macrosocial determinants of health, this chapter provides a new way of looking into how far-reaching the effects of the EU are on public health determinants, and the limited consideration of health impacts in those policy areas that indirectly affect public health.

To understand the EU's involvement in public health and the reasons it struggles to prioritise public health and wellbeing, it is useful to link

C. Godziewski, *The Politics of Health Promotion*, Palgrave Studies in Science, Knowledge and Policy, https://doi.org/10.1007/978-3-030-97870-9_5

the particular issue of health to the broader debate around institutional constellations that favour an economic Europe over a social one. As mentioned in a previous chapter, some have explained the lack of a public health vision as being reflective of the fact that the EU, ultimately, is a market-creating endeavour that promotes first and foremost economic integration. In turn, mechanisms through which the involvement of the EU in public health tends to occur is via the Single Market, and, more recently, via EU economic governance and the fiscal coordination of member states.

As the HiAP agenda is driven by a principle of mainstreaming, institutional space for health consideration needs to be critically assessed in soft-, hard- and meta-regulatory governance spaces. EU involvement in health promotion has traditionally been thought of in terms of (softly) regulating NCD risk factors. While this needs to be taken into consideration, it is not sufficient: health promotion also needs to be located and mainstreamed in entirely different spaces, such as fiscal governance. This is very much the point of HiAP. Yet the links between policy areas like trade, economic governance, foreign policy and health are rarely considered, and HiAP can become pragmatically focused on easier win–win situations (Baum et al., 2019). The proximal/distal health promotion relevance 'scale', with 'distal' spaces representing the macrosocial determinants of health and 'proximal' spaces pertaining to behavioural health promotion, tends to loosely align with the soft/hard dichotomy of EU governance. By 'policies addressing proximal determinants of health', I mean those initiatives targeted at behaviour and choice, including health education, information, nudging policies and incentives for food reformulation. These are often (though not always) governed in 'softer' ways. Macrosocial determinants of health, on the other hand, often remain shaped in hard(er) and more 'overarching'[1] governance areas. The hardest EU governance areas, and those that pertain to the overarching vision of the EU, tend to be those with the least *perceived* relevance to health promotion. This chapter highlights and contrasts these differential dynamics as illustrations of how EU constitutional asymmetry operates in relation to taking up HiAP, and how constitutional asymmetry precludes an understanding

[1] What is meant here with 'overarching', is meta-regulatory governance. Meta-regulatory governance is not classifiable as hard or soft per se (it tends to be a combination of both), but it shapes the institution at a both high and deep level.

of HiAP as being about macrosocial determinants of health. Considering the mantra coined under the Juncker Commission—according to which the EU needs to be 'bigger and more ambitious on big things, and smaller and more modest on small things' (European Commission, 2014a, p. 2)—we can see how difficult it would be for a HiAP shift to take place in an institutional context where economic growth is systematically privileged over societal wellbeing and health,[2] through an institutional architecture skewed in favour of negative integration over positive integration. Bearing in mind the breadth of the scope of this analysis, this chapter uses a selection of examples from different areas and types of EU governance that are all relevant for health promotion mainstreaming. Table 5.1 explains the rationale for the chosen examples, their position on the hard-, soft- and meta-regulatory governance categorisation, and their relevance to health promotion mainstreaming.

The remainder of this chapter follows the organisation outlined in the table above. Each example listed above is first described, before analysing the scope for HiAP it offers. Overall, this chapter highlights the EU constitutional asymmetry in relation to HiAP and in particular in relation to the need to adopt a radically broad vision for health promotion.

5.1 HiAP and EU Public Health Promotion

Following Greer's first face of EU involvement in public health, we will begin by looking at EU public health promotion policies. Public health promotion policies, which in this case refer to policies specifically designed to improve what is commonly referred to as the population's 'lifestyle' (the promotion of physical activity and healthy nutrition), are situated largely in the realm of EU soft governance. Their main purpose is to foster voluntary commitment and voluntary collaboration to achieve a stated aim like promoting healthy 'lifestyles'. Arguably the two best examples of EU policy in this area are the High Level Group on nutrition and physical activity (HLG) and the EU Platform for Action on Diet, Physical Activity and Health (EU Diet Platform). The HLG is a type of OMC-like space that brings together member states to collaborate and learn from each other in the field of NCDs prevention and health promotion. The EU Diet Platform is a multistakeholder platform aimed at incentivising private

[2] The two do not necessarily always preclude each other, but the prioritisation of one over the other has implications and entails trade-offs.

Table 5.1 Chapter overview: exploring EU constitutional asymmetry

Type of governance - soft/hard	Governance area	Policy or 'tool' (broadly defined)	Analytical purpose of example chosen	Type of health determinant at stake
Soft governance (NMG)	Public health promotion and NCD prevention	The EU Platform for action on Diet, Physical Activity and Health	The scope for HiAP in the soft governance approach to health promotion which relies on industry self-regulation and corporate social responsibility actions	*Individual behaviour/direct risk factors* **Proximal**
Soft governance (NMG)	Public health promotion and NCD prevention	The High Level Group for Nutrition and Physical Activity	The scope for HiAP in the soft governance approach to health promotion which facilitates voluntary knowledge exchange and mutual learning between member states (OMC)	*Individual behaviour/direct risk factors*
Hard governance	Single Market Regulation	The Audio-Visual Media Services Directive	The scope for health promotion mainstreaming in a non-health Single Market regulation	*Individual behaviour/direct risk factors*
Hard governance	The Common Agricultural Policy	The 'post-2020 CAP' Reforms	The scope for health promotion mainstreaming in the largest EU redistributive policy	*Food system*
Hard governance	EU economic governance	The European Semester	The scope for health promotion mainstreaming in the EU economic governance	*Socioeconomic inequities*
Meta-regulatory governance		The Better Regulation Agenda	The scope for HiAP in the EC's impact assessment and stakeholder consultation regime	*Governance processes and rationality*
Meta-regulatory governance		DG SANTE 2016-2020 Strategy	The scope for HiAP in the context of collegiality and the Commission priority streamlining	*Political vision and rationality* **Distal**

and public stakeholders to commit to healthy lifestyle promoting actions. This section will take look at both policy tools and evaluate the scope they offer in terms of reflecting a HiAP approach.

The EU Platform for Action on Diet, Physical Activity and Health

The EU Diet Platform is a multistakeholder Platform which brings together NGOs and industry to make commitments towards reducing the burden of diet and physical activity related NCDs. Members include representatives of the private sector, such as the advertising-, food-

and retail industry. They also include representatives of health advocacy groups and NGOs, as well as members of medical and paramedical profession groups and a few research-focused associations (European Commission, 2018a). Platform members are required to commit to concrete actions, referred to as 'commitments', in the field of healthy nutrition and physical activity.

> The idea is that, led by the Commission, the platform will provide an example of coordinated action on this problem by different parts of society that will encourage national, regional or local initiatives across Europe. (European Commission, n.d.a)

Platform members can be representatives of umbrella organisations and may not necessarily have commitments directly, in which case commitments need be made by at least one of their own members. This is an important point insofar as some industry members represent a very large number of very large companies (e.g. FoodDrinkEurope or the Union of EU soft drinks associations [UNESDA]). Critics of the Platform have argued that, due to the inclusion of such large umbrella organisations representing a large number of large food corporations, and the amount of resources that the private sector can dedicate to the Platform compared to the voluntary sector, the Platform is very much dominated by the private sector, despite the number of official members being more or less balanced between private and voluntary sector. Additionally and quite fundamentally, issues of inherent conflict of interest arise when positioning the food industry as a norm setter and policy influencer in reducing the diet-related NCD burden (Garde et al., 2017).

These weaknesses and critical issues have led to the recent withdrawal *en masse* of NGOs from the EU Diet Platform, much in the same way they withdrew from the twin multistakeholder Platform for Alcohol policy, the 'Alcohol Forum' in 2015 (EurActive, 2015; European Heart Network et al., 2019a). The withdrawal from the EU Diet Platform came after DG SANTE failed to respond to a call from these NGOs for 'an urgent, profound and meaningful overhaul to improve the Platform's outcomes' (European Heart Network et al., 2019a, p. 1; 2019b).

To analyse the (in)compatibility of the EU Diet Platform with the HiAP idea, it is worth looking at the kinds of results the EU Diet

Platform produces. Platform commitments tend to revolve around traditional public health initiatives that conceptualise healthy behaviour as an individual responsibility:

- 'The active commitments focus on six activity areas:
- Advocacy and information exchange (21 commitments);
- Composition of foods (reformulation), availability of healthy food options, portion sizes (18 commitments);
- Consumer information, including labelling (12 commitments);
- Education, including lifestyle modification (33 commitments);
- Marketing and advertising (14 commitments); and
- Physical activity promotion (11 commitments)' (European Commission, 2016a, p. 1).

It is perhaps not surprising to observe that these are the kinds of commitments taken by what are predominantly processed food and soft drink companies. These types of commitments are not designed to reflect an understanding of or a willingness to consider the complex political and ideological determinants that underlie the NCD burden, which are rooted in (health) inequities. Instead, these activities neatly fit the individual responsibility narrative of public health according to which healthy eating and healthy moving is largely a matter of educating people. The EU Diet Platform, in turn, nudges corporations to act responsibly—if they wish—in a way that facilitates individuals to do the same. Corporate social responsibility ultimately might serve the corporation's self-interest in various ways: to avoid future regulation and to position themselves as norm-setters, thereby increasing their power in society, among other reasons (see, e.g., Garriga & Melé, 2004). In the case of healthy diet promotion, the corporate social responsibility agenda of food and drink industries serves to reinforce individual responsibility narratives as well (Herrick, 2009). Many interviewees, including some EC officials,[3] expressed their rejection of the 'individual responsibility narrative' in public health and in relation to NCDs, and were aware of the links between that discourse, industry self-regulation and neoliberal capitalism. Many health policymakers seem to be aware of the need to address structural determinants of health, and the need for approaches like HiAP which

[3] Source: interviewees 3, 8, 12, 13, 20, 26, 31.

consider policy areas that shape socioeconomic inequities. Policy-wise, however, governance tools like the Platform do not reflect this understanding. The prominence of the EU Diet Platform had been decreasing for a while, and even more so since the withdrawal of many NGOs. The frequency of meetings has decreased, and the online presence of the Platform on EU website has also been cut back.

This tension between HiAP awareness and elaborating/maintaining policies like the EU Diet Platform reflects a tendency for policies and initiatives to revert to individual behaviour modification. This tendency has been identified in the literature as the 'lifestyle drift' (Powell et al., 2017; Williams & Fullagar, 2019). The 'lifestyle drift' is a phenomenon in public health policy defined as 'the tendency for policy to start off recognizing the need for action on upstream social determinants of health inequalities only to drift downstream to focus largely on individual lifestyle factors' (Popay et al., 2010, p. 148). Baum and Fisher (2014) provide an overview of the multiple explanatory dimensions of the lifestyle drift—historical, ideological technical and interest-driven. In terms of historical and ideological factors, they clearly link lifestyle drift with the deployment and consolidation of neoliberal rationality (Baum & Fisher, 2014). Carey et al. (2017) have applied a framework of the sociology of social problems to explain the lifestyle drift. Their model is based on the idea that social problems are considered 'negative residue' of dominant political processes. The politics of placing a problem within or outside the social sphere is key, as the exclusion of problems outside the social sphere (and into either the private, personal sphere, or the medical, pathological one, or one that is limited to particular groups of people deemed 'abnormal') is a way to obscure the problematic consequences of a particular political system or a particular ideology. They used this sociological model to argue that the way in which obesity as an issue is placed outside the public sphere and is framed as a problem affecting mostly people from vulnerable socio-economic background (Carey et al., 2017). Once a problem is framed in such a way, the route is paved for interventions targeted at disciplining and/or saving 'at-risk groups' and thinking of health inequities as a gap to fill by targeting policies at poorer people (Carey et al., 2017; M. Douglas, 2015; Smith, 2013; Wilkinson & Pickett, 2010). When asked about the Platform's potential to address inequalities, the response of one policymaker interviewee illustrated this rationale that action on inequalities is about upward-filling of a gap:

> I think the Platform can develop ideas for improving approaches for vulnerable population. One example [...] is the idea of introducing quality criteria for food banks. Food banks are not necessarily carrying the poorest quality food but might not be in a position to pay enough attention to the nutritional quality of the food. I think it's quite possible to look at the aspects of social inequalities within the Platform and indeed the intention is not to improve the health of the ones at the top, but to improve the health of the ones at the bottom. (Quote from interviewee 29)

This is a common conflation between inequality and poverty, which, following the sociology of social problems model, places the issue of NCDs in the realm of the private. For example, the suggestion to improve the food quality of food banks is about changing food banks, as well as changing the behaviour of poor people by facilitating their access to healthier food. In no way is this kind of policy targeted at reducing the number of people who would need food banks in the first place.

The point is not that the EU Diet Platform should address the macrosocial determinants of NCDs, but that the EU Diet Platform cannot address and even *actively deters from addressing* structural determinants of NCDs, because of the very nature and essential characteristics of that tool. It is incompatible with the essence of the HiAP idea at EU level insofar as its rationale places the responsibility for HiAP away from EU policymakers and away from policy areas that *appear* to be unrelated to health and onto 'responsible corporations' and 'responsible citizens'. This undermines the whole point that HiAP is about understanding and addressing the indirect, macrosocial determinants of health situated precisely in non-health policy areas and moving away from conflating health promotion with individual behaviour modification.[4]

The High-Level Group on Nutrition and Physical Activity

The HLG was created in 2007, at the same time as the EC published its obesity strategy (European Commission, 2007). The group is composed of EU and European Free Trade Association (EFTA) member states government representatives who are involved on this particular public

[4] For a discussion on how the meaning of HiAP itself has been redefined to include an emphasis on multistakeholder involvement, see Chapter 7.

health issue at home. The role of the HLG is defined by the Commission as follows:

> [...] The group
>
> - Enables governments to share health and economic analysis, policy ideas and best practices and develop common approaches;
> - Works on priorities such as improving food products recipes, reducing children's exposure to marketing of foods high in fat, salt and sugars, physical activity, labelling and public procurement of food;
> - Enhances contact between governments and the EU Platform for action on diet, physical activity and health, so that relevant collaboration with and between stakeholders can take place.
> - Facilitates the sharing of evidence, data and best practices for policy makers;
> - Identifies research gaps and supports health in all policies;
> - Works on reducing health inequalities (European Commission, n.d.b)

The overwhelming opinion of HLG members on the group was positive.[5] The opportunities that the HLG offers were very much valued, including the possibilities to go abroad and learn about the implementation of particular policies or ways of working in a different member state.[6] In the past, the group had been presented by the EC website as an opportunity to foster dialogue between governments and the EU Diet Platform. However, none of the HLG members interviewed were actively supporting the idea of promoting more proximity between them and the EU Diet Platform, with some of them explicitly criticising that.[7] One interviewee stressed that the HLG was a space in which attempts were being made to really put HiAP at the centre, including by the EC.[8] The HLG was also perceived by some members as a very useful lever to raise

[5] Source: interviewees 15, 17, 18, 19, and 27.

[6] Source: interviewees 18 and 19.

[7] Source: interviewees 17 and 18.

[8] Source: interviewee 27.

public health issues on their respective national agendas.[9] The informal, less tangible, social perks of being a group with common interests and expertise that meets regularly was also raised as a very valuable dimension of the HLG.[10]

Another concrete example of the usefulness of the HLG portrayed in one interview was the pivotal role it played in the inclusion of the health and nutrition related marketing restrictions in the AVMSD. One interviewee described how it would not have been possible to coordinate a reaction on this issue from health ministries across member states if it hadn't been for the HLG and the fact that, thanks to the group, they knew each other and could get in touch easily and rapidly:

> When they started negotiating these parts that covered food marketing, and I noticed that the text they were proposing did not include the food and health related issues that the HLG had emphasised. So, I sent the message to my colleagues in the HLG saying 'Have you seen this?!' [...] And there was immediate reaction: in two days they'd contacted their colleagues in their relevant ministries. So, it can work as a kind of catalyst. (quoted from interviewee 27)

As seen above, supporting HiAP is an officially stated aim of the HLG, and HLG members are keen to see this group as an opportunity to work towards implementing HiAP in their respective member states and through influencing EU legislation. But how effective can a tool like the HLG be with respect to fostering a normatively meaningful HiAP along the lines of a radically broad understanding of health promotion? In other words, is the HLG a radical 'game-changer' that can bring about structural change towards prioritising societal wellbeing?

Even though it is not defined as an OMC, in some respects the HLG is similar to an OMC: it shares OMC core principles like the fostering of voluntary collaboration among member states through knowledge and best practices exchange. Much work has criticised the OMC on various fronts: some provide critical accounts of the (lack of) democratic legitimacy of these NMGs, and of the OMC in particular (De la Porte & Nanz, 2004; Kohler-Koch & Finke, 2007; Kröger, 2007; Radulova, 2007; Smismans, 2008). Others have argued that the OMC, as a tool

[9] Source: interviewees 17, 18, and 19.

[10] Source: interviewees 18 and 19.

of the Lisbon agenda for promoting growth and competitiveness, has reshaped the problematisation of social policy towards equipping responsible individuals to face modern labour market challenges, rather than protecting the solidarity-based mechanisms of traditional social policy (Parker, 2008). Despite its 'soft' and voluntary nature, the OMC has been effective at what Bruno et al., (2006, p. 532) call 'cognitive and normative harmonisation of national policies [that] disciplines the processes of Europeanization, by regulating governmental policy-making in a conceptual and pragmatic way, which conforms to the "management spirit"'.

However, the HLG also differs from the social OMC, most importantly in the benchmarking and monitoring of member states' progress on agreed upon goals. The HLG did set out a voluntary framework with benchmarks and targets for member states who want to act on food reformulation, specifically saturated fats, added sugar and salt (European Commission, 2008, 2011, 2012, 2015b). However, the purpose of such benchmarking is not directly related to the EC overarching agenda in the way that the social OMC is (see: Borrás & Jacobsson, 2004; De la Porte & Pochet, 2012; Shore, 2011). Consequently, it is not formally linked to the EU's economic governance through the European Semester. The HLG is not, as Bruno et al., (2006, p. 529) 'subordinated to the Broad Economic Policy Guidelines' in the quite the same direct way as real OMCs. In theory, this could allow more freedom to come up with radical suggestions to implement HiAP. In practice, however, and in the grand scheme of things, the agency and scope of the HLG remains limited and is unlikely to bring about radical change on its own. The HLG's work remains largely concerned with proximal determinants of health, such as food reformulation, even though the more recently officially added themes like supporting HiAP and reducing health inequalities might indicate an attempt—at least by the more critical members—to act upon macrosocial determinants of health. As long as it is limited to proximal determinants, the HLG might enjoy relative operational freedom. At the same time, however, the group is unlikely to carry enough weight to take HiAP further and adopt a radically broad approach to health promotion. This suspicion is based on the description interviewees gave of the process and the amount of work invested to include health in the AVMSD, and the outcome it ultimately led to (see separate section on AVMSD below).

5.2 HiAP and the EU Single Market

This section moves on to the potential for HiAP to be implemented in a non-health Single Market-specific issue. While it echoes Greer's second face of EU involvement in health, it is different insofar as this section is not about how Single Market regulations directly affect healthcare, but about the extent to which indirect effects of non-health Single Market regulations on health can be taken into consideration. When asked about a Single Market, non-health policy which illustrates an attempt to mainstream HiAP in relation to NCD prevention and health promotion in the EC, some interviewees mentioned the AVMSD.[11] The case of the AVMSD and the efforts to include health-related considerations in it was also brought up when discussing the role of the HLG.

The Audio-Visual Media Services Directive

In 2015/2016, the AVMSD underwent the REFIT process. REFIT is a tool of the Better Regulation Agenda to assess whether EU regulations are still up-to-date and do not cause an unnecessary burden on EU businesses and citizens (European Commission, 2017b). The public consultation on the directive addressed the issue of adequate consumer protection (European Commission, 2015c, p. 5). In 2016, the EC published a proposal for a revised AVMSD, in which it stated that it aimed to strike a balance between promoting competitiveness and protecting consumers (European Commission, 2016b, p. 12). In terms of protecting consumers from advertisement of unhealthy foods and alcohol, the proposal suggested strengthening self-regulatory and co-regulatory codes of conduct. However, evidence of the efficiency of industry self-regulation in the food and alcohol industry is weak (Moodie et al., 2013; Ronit & Jensen, 2014; Thornley et al., 2010). The European Public Health Alliance was one of the EU public health advocacy groups who used the REFIT cycle as an opportunity to actively campaign for a stronger inclusion of public health concerns in the AVMSD, in particular regarding restricting advertisement of unhealthy foods to children; excluding alcohol and unhealthy food ('high fat, sugar, salt' foods) from product placement and sponsorships; and allowing adequate regulatory space for member states on public health grounds (European Public

[11] Source: interviewees 13, 20 and 28.

Health Alliance, 2016a, 2016b, 2017). As mentioned above, the HLG also worked to include a stronger health basis in the AVMSD. The revision of the AVMSD was not unanimously seen as successful from a public health standpoint, and some of the health advocates interviewed expressed their frustration at the limited scope of the public health-related provisions in the proposal, as well as the EP's stance vis-à-vis the proposal.[12]

> A couple of MEPs were supportive but overwhelmingly [we faced] a brick wall. We had much more traction with member states on that particular issue. I think the reason for all this resistance was that the dossier wasn't dealt with by health attachés but by culture attachés [...]. I've never encountered such resistance like in the AVMSD. [...] We were a bit naive as well, because we later realised that asking them to stop advertising alcohol and junk food between 6am and 11pm was basically asking them to dismantle the whole system upon which their profit-making is based on. We didn't realise that we just blindly went in. That might be why we weren't successful. (quoted from interviewee 20)

Arguably, the EP's amendments and amendment proposals,[13] which revolved around encouraging industry self- and co-regulation to limit advertisement of unhealthy foods and alcohol, further weakened any pressure that could be put on the industry. The EP proposed to replace the reference to WHO nutrient profile guidelines with references to the EU Pledge[14] and the EU Diet Platform. They also proposed to replace the term 'with a significant children's audience' to 'content aimed at a children's audience' (European Parliament, 2017, pp. 79–102, in particular see amendment 14, p. 88), which would have narrowed the scope of

[12] Source: interviewees 13 and 20.

[13] In the EU legislative process, both the Council and the EP follow consultation procedures and add amendments to the initial proposal, which will then again be voted on. If after the second reading no agreement is found, the proposal undergoes a conciliation procedure, where it can ultimately end up being accepted or rejected. The procedure varies for the adoption of the EU budget and in certain other cases (see: Bache et al., 2015).

[14] The EU Pledge is an initiative led by food and beverage companies. It establishes norms and voluntary guidelines on responsible advertising to children. It is supposed 'to support parents in making the right diet and lifestyle choices for their children' (See EU Pledge website: https://eu-pledge.eu/).

the directive. The final text adopted in November 2018 refers to 'children's programmes' (European Union, 2018). The new AVMSD was passed on 14 November 2018, and in the end, it does include more explicit references to advertisement and product placement of unhealthy foods and alcohol than the 2010 version: the two main changes are that it now forbids product placement in children's programmes, and more explicitly encourages member states to foster effective industry self- and co-regulation (European Union, 2018, p. L303/73; European Parliament, 2019).

The case of the fight to include health concerns in the AVMSD is illustrative of the difficulty of generating positive integration and implementing HiAP. The regulatory process is such that it is difficult to accommodate HiAP, echoing what Scharpf conceptualises as negative and positive integration. While it now includes a line that mentions saturated fatty acids and some marketing restrictions, the struggles that were faced to achieve this relatively small step shows the absence of vision for health and wellbeing at the centre of EU governance. Hard work may well have been done to include a sentence referring to public health in a particular policy, but this does not mean that the EU, including the EC, has undergone a shift in vision which now puts societal wellbeing and health above economic interests and growth. The dominant view remains that, in the process of integrating the Single Market, these kinds of health aspects should not be regulated. This is in line with the imperative of preserving the freedom of the market as much as possible, and it is reflected in the prevailing and re-affirmed position to first and foremost encourage industry self-regulation. Notwithstanding that the AVMSD case represents an attempt to implement HiAP, the relative success of this attempt is very much limited to one small technical aspect of HiAP. But it is not accompanied by a more diffuse normative change towards HiAP.

5.3 HiAP and the Common Agricultural Policy

The CAP is the oldest and remained for a long time the only, EU redistributive policy (Ackrill et al., 2008). The CAP's history dates to the 1960s, as part of the broader integration plan to create a common market (Garzon, 2006; Walls et al., 2016). It was created to ensure stable food supply. However, flawed the initial price support system was, its logic was a reflection of the post-war period and the immediate concern with preventing food shortage. As such, some have argued that the CAP was inherently a public health measure as well as a market integration measure (European Public Health Alliance, 2016c, p. 5). There are obvious reasons why the CAP is a policy with very strong relevance to HiAP, including in specific relation to health promotion and NCD prevention: poor diets, alcohol and tobacco consumption are important determinants of NCDs, and agricultural policies play a very important role in configuring the availability and price of these products within the EU Single Market and abroad. Until now, the CAP's objectives revolved around five key principles:

- support farmers and improve agricultural productivity, ensuring a stable supply of affordable food
- safeguard European Union (EU) farmers to make a reasonable living
- help tackle climate change and the sustainable management of natural resources
- maintain rural areas and landscapes across the EU
- keep the rural economy alive by promoting jobs in farming, agri-foods industries and associated sectors (European Commission, n.d.c).

Important issues remain in terms of the health sensitivity (as well as environmental sustainability) of the budget distribution. Over the last decades, taking health and environmental protection into account in the CAP has proven a political minefield. With the current system dominated by direct payments, the CAP disproportionately benefits a small group of large, richer and intensive farms. The post-Eurozone crisis proposed cuts to the CAP were shaped in part by the powerful farmer lobby who proposed to save money mainly from the environmental measures and rural development pillar (Pe'er et al., 2019; Roederer-Rynning & Matthews, 2019). The CAP money in 2005 predominantly supported food groups of which consumption needs to be decreased (for health as well as environmental sustainability reasons), as well as harmful products like wine and tobacco (Birt et al., 2007, cited in European Public Health Alliance, 2016c, p. 9).

The Post-2020 CAP Reforms

With the growing public outrage about the climate emergency and the unsustainability (both environmentally and socially) of the global food system, the CAP is under increasing societal pressure to respond to modern food-related challenges, including the health aspects of agricultural practices and food production. According to a Eurobarometer study (cited in: Pe'er et al., 2019, p. 449), 92% of non-farmers and 64% of farmers agree that the CAP should do more to address environmental challenges such as the climate crisis. The CAP is set to be reformed again for the post-2020 period, and some health NGOs have been advocating for reforms that more strongly reflect the linkages between agriculture and health (European Public Health Alliance, 2016c). Prior to the pandemic, the EC had released a set of proposals for a reformed CAP with new objectives. Overall, these were mainly presented as a response to the need to modernise and simplify in a way that gives more autonomy and flexibility to member states and farmers (European Commission, 2017c, 2018b, 2019a). The new objectives of the policy, while expressed vaguely, are to be revised in a way that better reflects the challenges of today. The last specific objective is explicitly to protect food and health quality (European Commission, 2018c, n.d.c).

Given these new objectives and the repeated emphasis put on issues like climate change and the link between public health and farming, could it be expected that the new CAP represents a 'HiAP-sensitive' reform? One interviewee from an EU health NGO (interviewed in 2018) pointed out that, while rhetorically it would be almost untenable not to pay attention to these so-called societal challenges, how this will be reflected in practice, is far from clear:

> It is very positive, because you say ok this policy has a social element, an environmental element, an economic element, a health element. That's something you'd expect from a holistic policy in principle. So, in principle it looks quite progressive. But a lot will depend on how member states are kept accountable to it. (quoted from interviewee 13)

Indeed, the first obvious shortcoming identified back in 2018/19 was the lack of clear mechanisms to enforce compliance with the newly listed goals (European Commission, 2018c, 2018d; European Public Health Alliance, 2018; Pe'er et al., 2019). The other strong emphasis, along with providing member states more flexibility and subsidiarity, is to make the CAP more results-oriented. To do so, the EC will resort to defining indicators that are supposed to measure how well a member state is performing. However, especially in the areas relevant to public health and environmental protection, the indicators tend to be limited to measuring the proportion of farms that have made various commitments, but it does not capture what Pe'er et al., (2019, p. 451) refer to as 'real impacts' (European Commission, 2018e). There was initially little concrete guidance about how the goals of promoting nutritious food, as well as reducing inequalities among farmers of different sizes, were supposed to be achieved (see: European Commission, 2018e, p. 6). The proportion of payment as direct payments—which have been consolidating social and environmental unsustainability—is increased, and the redistributive mechanisms directed at rebalancing inequities and help smaller farms 'remain weak' (Pe'er et al., 2019, p. 450). Similarly to the post-Eurozone crisis budget cuts, the expected Brexit-induced budgetary decrease is also likely to affect the second CAP pillar funding (i.e. funding related to rural development, which includes much of the environmental and social sustainability aspects) disproportionately (Roederer-Rynning & Matthews, 2019).

While rhetorically, there may well be increased consideration for food and farming as closely linked to health, and health understood broadly in a way that includes environmental wellbeing and animal welfare, in practice there is still more to be done for these ideas to be meaningfully reflected in action. The absence of a meaningful environmental, economic and social sustainability-oriented mindset of these reforms raises serious doubts with respect to how much improvement—if any at all—they will be able to achieve (Pe'er et al., 2019). Another key question mark is how the EU will make sure member states comply with these new goals, especially when the accent of the reform is put on increased subsidiarity, and increased freedom for member states to adapt, adjust and interpret the CAP according to their national contexts.

In 2020, the Commission published further strategic documents aimed at aligning the CAP with the European Green Deal, and specifically with the 'Farm to Fork' strategy on sustainable food systems, as well as the 'Biodiversity strategy' (European Commission, 2020a, 2020b). These contain concrete action plans on how to make the food system more health-sensitive and the CAP more environmentally sustainable. The EC also published a fact sheet laying out its ambitions and action plan and outlining the EP and the Council's position vis-a-vis all the individual points (European Commission, 2020c). It will be interesting to see how the CAP develops in the future, especially in the context of the European Green Deal and the acute quadruple crisis (environmental, social, economic and health) we are now facing.

5.4 HiAP and EU Fiscal Governance

So far, we have looked at the space for HiAP in selected examples of health promotion soft governance, in a non-health Single Market directive in the frame of the REFIT process, and the CAP. Now we move on to explore the space for HiAP in EU fiscal governance, in particular pertaining to the relationship between EU fiscal coordination and social policy. This is related to what Greer calls the third (most recent) face of EU involvement in health. This section takes as a starting point the streamlining dynamics between the European Structural and Investment Fund (ESIF) and EU fiscal governance mechanisms, in particular the European Semester. It then reflects on the broader relevance of EU fiscal governance to macrosocial determinants of health, re-emphasising the need to look beyond impacts solely on national health systems, and towards a recognition that all measures influencing public spending are relevant to public health.

Investment in Health and the European Semester

Prior to the COVID-19 pandemic and the tools set up specifically to promote post-pandemic economic recovery, the second largest EU budget expenditure (after the CAP) was the ESIF. Health-related investments under the ESIF have been said to represent HiAP in action (Merkel, 2010). Over the 2007–2013 period, 1.5% of the structural funds were invested in health infrastructure, which amounts to just under EUR 5.2 billion (European Commission, 2016c, p. 10). It is, in absolute terms, much more than the expenditures under the Health Programme (HP), which amounted to EUR 321.5 million for the 2008–2014 period (European Commission, 2015d, p. 3). This sum is also limited to health infrastructure expenditures and does not include other investments that have a positive impact on health indirectly. The 2014–2020 ESIF programming period saw an increase in health-related investment (an increase of what falls into the classification of health-related investment). Based on an analysis of the ESIF projects approved by August 2017 for the 2014–2020 programming period, (and more specifically within the three sub-funds relevant to health[15]) over 7000 projects had relevance to health and more than EUR 8 billion were spent on health (European Commission, 2019b, p. 19). One of the key evolutions of the ESIF for health is the move away from favouring investment in large infrastructure projects (what is called 'hard' investment) and towards investment in human capital and resources, training and life-long learning (referred to as 'soft' investment).

The other important way the ESIF has evolved is that, for investments in health, it is now closely related to the European Semester process, and member states who benefit from ESIF money and wish to invest in health—which is the case in largest part for Eastern European countries and, to some extent, Southern European countries—need to make use of this money as part of a broader strategic framework aligned with Semester recommendations on health systems (European Commission, 2019b). What this means is that this EU redistributive tool at the disposal of member states wishing to use it to invest in health is now increasingly streamlined with the EU fiscal and economic governance.

Given the relevance of the ESIF to HiAP, it is worth exploring what the increased streamlining of the ESIF with the European Semester might mean in practice. Out of the various EU fiscal governance reforms, the Semester has been perceived as the least opaque and rigid one, one that might potentially be malleable enough to be directed in a more socially progressive direction. At the same time, there is concern with the Semester's intrusion—through health systems CSR—into national health systems, an area which has always been vehemently guarded to remain in the hands of member states (Azzopardi-Muscat & Brand, 2014; EuroHealthNet, 2018; Zeitlin & Vanhercke, 2014). Indeed, it has been argued that health care systems are increasingly becoming a shared competence, as the Semester now attributes health-related CSR (Azzopardi-Muscat et al., 2015). The emphasis of these CSR is put on (financial) sustainability and cost-effectiveness, more than a framing in terms of the social pillar to combat poverty and social exclusion. This represents a clear instance of constitutional asymmetry.

The rationale for the involvement of the EC in member states' health systems through the health-specific CSR is that health systems represent

[15] The European Regional Development Fund (ERDF), the European Social Fund (ESF) and the Cohesion Fund (CF). It excludes the European Agricultural Fund for Rural Development; and the European Maritime and Fisheries Fund.

an important part of public spending, and that for the EU's economic stability in this post-crisis period, it is important to ensure that member states' health systems are fiscally sustainable:

> Modern health systems need to remain accessible and effective while pursuing long-term sustainability. To do this, they have to remain fiscally sustainable. The Commission supports member states in this work, providing analysis and forecasts, and recommending reforms as part of the European Semester process [...] EU health systems have not coped equally well with the economic crisis and some have had to implement major and sometimes painful reforms in a very short time. (European Commission, 2014b, p. 10).

Concretely, the Semester's health specific recommendations are oriented towards, among other things, promoting eHealth, mHealth and performance assessments (European Commission, 2017d, p. 9). This is seen as the innovative direction that will help fiscal sustainability of health systems (European Commission, 2017d). Pensions and healthcare are the two largest public expenditures in the EU (European Commission, 2016d), and the two are seen as relatedly growing given the ageing population. Generally speaking, the Semester's advice in terms of pensions seems to be to decrease pension benefits and/or revise the age of retirement. It is worth reflecting upon the coherence of these kinds of policy direction, as regarding their potential impact on the financial burden of the ageing population on the healthcare system. The current involvement of the Semester in the area of health has little to do with population health per se; rather, it is about ensuring fiscal sustainability of the health systems and making health systems more cost-effective (Azzopardi-Muscat et al., 2015).

Economic priorities are cemented in the conditionalities for accessing the ESIF. This leaves little space for HiAP and relates more to the constitutional asymmetry which systematically prioritises economic growth over social wellbeing. As a result of the toughened EU fiscal control mechanisms elaborated after the Eurozone crisis, the EC and the Council now have powerful tools to shape member states' public spending. Chapter Six will provide a deeper analysis into the normative paradigms that drive the Semester's involvement in health, and the frames through which this takes place.

5.5 HiAP and EU Meta-Regulation

The last section of this chapter is concerned with the scope for HiAP beyond specific governance sectors, and in terms of overarching governance logic, that is, in terms of meta-regulation. This governance aspect does not fit with Greer's faces of EU involvement in health, because it does not necessarily fit with the model of neo-functionalist spill over into the field of public health and health care. Starting from the notion that HiAP is a concept that needs to be taken up across the board—mainstreamed—it is important to evaluate the scope for HiAP in the EC's meta-regulatory landscape. The elements analysed in this section are the ones briefly introduced under the relevant section in a previous chapter: Better Regulation and the collegiality principle.

Better Regulation: Impact Assessment and Stakeholder Consultation Regime

One of the most important aspects of Better Regulation is the need to undertake extensive integrated IA. IA goes hand in hand with stakeholder consultations, as the process includes them at multiple stages, and relies on information provided by stakeholders (European Commission, 2009, 2015a). Once political validation by the relevant Commissioner and Vice-President(s) has been obtained, an inter-service group (ISG) made up of officials from various DGs on whose area the proposal is likely to impact, is created. The ISG is responsible for drafting the evaluation roadmap and inception IA. At this early stage, the process normally includes a plan to consult stakeholders: they have four weeks to provide input (European Commission, 2017a). A Regulatory Scrutiny Board also issues opinions on the IA, fitness checks and evaluations, separately from the other DGs. All feedback must be taken into careful consideration. The IA is then re-evaluated and published for another eight weeks of stakeholder feedback (European Commission, 2017a).

The integrated IA is supposed to consider not only economic, but also social and environmental impacts. The 2017 Better Regulation guidelines include a section on assessing health impact. While it does mention, at several stages, the existence and importance of non-monetary estimations of health impacts, and the requirement that health impacts should be presented in both monetary and non-monetary terms (such as the number of life years lost) the largest part of the guideline section focuses on monetary estimates (how numbers of life years lost translate into lost productivity, for example). The limitations of these measurements are acknowledged in the guidelines (European Commission, 2017a). In terms of stakeholder consultation, the EC has shown increasing commitment, over the past few decades, to engaging more with civil society groups and NGOs in domains not usually associated with civil society, and to increasing transparency (Kohler-Koch & Finke, 2007).

How, then, does HiAP fit into this meta-regulatory picture? HIA could be seen as the logical 'HiAP dimension' of Better Regulation. They have been considered with much enthusiasm by some researchers and in particular one health advocate interviewed,[16] provided HIA can be perfected and taken seriously (Kemm, 2006).

However, the process of heavy IA and thorough stakeholder consultation has been argued to be strongly skewed in favour of business interests. The remainder of this section critically evaluates the scope for a HiAP rationale at the meta-regulatory level of Better Regulation. The most striking example in the literature on corporate interest permeating the Better Regulation agenda is the tobacco industry's effort to shape and use the IA process to its advantage (Costa et al., 2014; Peeters et al., 2016; Smith et al., 2009, 2010a, 2015). These investigations reveal how the shift towards Better Regulation was actively pursued by the tobacco industry to neutralise the threat posed to them by the precautionary principle. The precautionary principle refers to the need and legitimacy for policymakers to intervene to prevent public health hazard if there are reasonable grounds to believe that a hazard would occur and result in severe or irreversible damage to public health. This principle applies even if there is no clear scientific consensus about the likelihood of the hazard occurring (see: Smith et al., 2015, p. 332). The tobacco industry reckoned that, if it succeeded in institutionalising a risk assessment, which the industry itself would play a considerable role in shaping, the regulatory landscape would shift from a cautious rationale to protect human health, to one in which 'new measures are not adopted unless they will achieve significant risk reduction at a reasonable cost, and [in which] new regulations and legislation are based on quantitative risk assessment' (Smith et al., 2015, p. 334).

[16] Source: interviewee 26.

To push its desired IA agenda, the tobacco industry hid behind the mobilisation of a coalition of businesses, which gave the impression of consensus across the private sector, and behind certain trusted Brussels think tanks such as the European Policy Centre. Calls for more transparency and dialogue also served the tobacco industry in placing itself in a privileged position to provide data and influence the policymaking process (Smith et al., 2015). Smith et al. (2010b) have outlined eight fundamental concerns about IAs and their ingrained bias in favour of industry. One of the concerns was that IAs, given the extent and time-consuming nature of this bureaucratic task, are often used to delay regulation[17] (Smith et al., 2010b). Delays can be achieved for example by invoking 'lack of evidence'. This tactic relates to the instrumentalisation of evidence and what Parkhurst (2017) refers to as 'technical bias' in evidence-based policymaking. This point was captured by one interviewee from an EU NGO:

> Impact assessment now has become much more complex. [...] It's also become a battle ground; so again [regarding] the most recent tobacco control directive. An impact assessment was done [...]. And then the industry lobbied against it, called it into question, complained to the impact assessment board in the EC. So the EC had to, they decided to commission not just one new impact assessment on the draft directive, but they commissioned 5 impact assessments. Which built in another 2, 3, 4 years delay. (quoted from interviewee 20)

Given all the considerations above, one can understandably be critical about the space for a HiAP rationality in the current Better Regulation context. HIA can be seen as the most technocratic interpretation of HiAP, and it can also be perceived to 'degenerate into a tokenistic "tick box" procedure' (Kemm, 2006, p. 202). Furthermore, HIA may not be adequate for national and international policy evaluation, as it was created mainly as a tool to evaluate smaller-scale projects at local levels (Koivusalo,

[17] The others pertain to the overreliance on simplified, aggregate monetary prediction which obscure uncertainties and complexities of policymaking and its effects, and which also obscures the nuances of varying distribution of impacts. They also note the problematic asymmetry of information resulting notably from relying on industry data to estimate the costs to business of an additional regulation, a cost which is easier to calculate than future societal benefits stemming from the regulation. They also highlight the problematic nature of the economic paradigm of for health and how it is perpetuated though the IA rationale.

2010). Importantly, HIA is no match for the integrated IA structurally biased in favour of private economic interests. Finally, and more fundamentally: A strong and protected precautionary principle reflects a HiAP rationality far better than the pursuit of a flawless HIA. This does not negate the value of researching health impacts and how to measure them, but it warns against the legitimisation of a system skewed against public health interests.

EC Collegiality and the DG SANTE Strategic Plan

EC decision-making is guided by the principle of collegiality. This means that decisions, such as new legislative proposals, need to be approved by the college of commissioners as a whole. At the suspicion that the voice of certain DGs, in the collegial space, carry more weight than others, one interviewee responded:

> I wouldn't say it's fair at all. It depends I think on the amount of evidence you have for a specific argument. [...] If you have that evidence [that a minimum pricing unit reduces alcohol harm to society] you're in a stronger position than if you don't have that evidence. It all boils down to how strong the evidence is. (quoted from interviewee 28)

This quote suggests that the collegiality principle is neutral, and that streamlining EC priorities through fostering this close collaboration leads to rational decision-making based on available evidence. In theory, then, one would expect that increased collegiality could offer the space to raise health on the agenda across DGs, and to facilitate HiAP. However, reinforced collegiality in the decision-making process has in certain cases meant that a DG's agency becomes more constrained. This is especially true for small DGs like SANTE. One MEP assistant explained how collegiality has meant a reduction in the number of proposals initiated by DG SANTE (a reduction in numbers of legislative and regulatory proposals is, after all, one of the most crucial goals of Better Regulation):

> [...] there's a different procedure now. Before, DG SANTE could just come up with ideas, with proposals. But now it has to undergo a cross... [sic] it has to be decided by the Commissioners from all different DGs, because of collegiality. A lot of initiatives have been stopped because of the new procedure. (quoted from interviewee 21)

The relatively recent increased number of invitations of health to the negotiating table also meant, according to one interviewee, that those supposed to represent health can easily become caught up in a dynamic of subordinating their own sector to the needs and imperative of other sectors. Arguably, this issue is visible in how the aims and goals of each DG have been aggressively streamlined towards EC overarching priorities: in the case of DG SANTE, the need to streamline Juncker priorities is reflected in the DG's strategic plan for 2016–2020 (European Commission, 2017e). The plan states that 'DG SANTE's primary objective is to contribute to jobs, growth, and investment in the EU' (p. 11), and that 'DG SANTE's ultimate goal is to achieve better conditions for trade: greater market access for EU exports at the same time as ensuring our food standards are not compromised on imports' (p. 28).

Throughout the document, the case for health is justified in terms of how it contributes to the Juncker priorities. In terms of growth and jobs, the narrative is one that stresses the health and care sector, as well as the food sector, as two very important parts of the economy. The justification for investment in health is that it can prevent large amounts of money getting lost to burdensome and expensive treatments of diseases, and that, therefore, the EU needs to invest in preventing diseases, as well as developing innovative solutions to absorb the costs of healthcare, such as e-health, m-health and telemedicine. In terms of competitiveness, the strategy speaks of promoting the internationally recognised 'safety brand' (p. 4) and remaining a world leader in the safety of products, such as foodstuffs, that move inside the Single Market. The way SANTE negotiates competitiveness and food safety, which at first sight can seem contradictory (insofar as competitiveness is associated with deregulation and safety is associated with regulation) is in terms of the 'EU brand' as being a world leading example of safety and trustworthiness (European Commission, 2017e). Key challenges for DG SANTE in the 2016–2020 period identified in the strategy include increasing cost-effectiveness, balancing safety and competitiveness, global health threats, making policymaking more evidence-based, and balancing consumer safety and industrial interests. Regarding industry interests, the strategy also proposes to intensify close collaboration with stakeholders. DG SANTE is also placed within a context of trade relations and identifies as one of its roles the promotion of trade relations, including through working towards removing SPS trade barriers with the United States. Interestingly, the burden of NCDs and health promotion only figure under the 'improving cost-efficiency' headline, and social determinants of health, HiAP or health inequities are not mentioned in the operating context.

The 2016–2020 Strategic Plan makes it very clear that population health is not the primary concern of Juncker's DG SANTE, but that health is merely an avenue to contributing to economic growth and competitiveness, which is aligned with the overarching EC priorities. While this does not preclude some very limited, technical instances of including health in non-health-related policy areas, for example in the form of calculating the financial impact of proposed policies on health systems, it does not allow for a normatively meaningful HiAP, given the way the EC and DG SANTE priorities are clearly stated.

5.6 Conclusion: An Unfavourable Institutional Context

This chapter has made the case that the EU institutional context is not particularly favourable for implementing HiAP in a normatively meaningful way. That the institutional setting of the EU is geared in favour of the free market and economic growth, and that therefore, it offers little scope for HiAP, is not surprising and concurs with the critical literature on EU health that situates the involvement of the EU in health within the constitutional asymmetry context and the neoliberal bias of the EU.

This chapter has contributed to this critical EU health literature with new empirical foci related to health promotion, rather than healthcare services and health systems, which tended to be the focus thus far. By taking a broad conceptualisation of health promotion, it has explored some of the institutional barriers to HiAP using examples from a large variety of EU governance aspects: it started with soft governance tools directly aimed at public health promotion and NCD prevention. Here, we looked at how the EU Diet Platform and its actions are symptomatic of the 'lifestyle drift' phenomenon, and how it contributes to perpetuating that phenomenon. Meanwhile, the OMC-like space for nutrition and physical activity, the HLG, while it is not subject to the same pressures as the social OMC, ends up having limited scope beyond action on proximal determinants of health, despite the enthusiasm and efforts of its members. In the 'hard governance' category, this chapter has provided examples of the lack of a HiAP vision in the Single Market (the AVMSD), the CAP reforms and EU fiscal governance. Yet all these governance areas are relevant to HiAP: the Single Market and the CAP shape the availability and prices of products, and all three areas have indirect implications on health through shaping socioeconomic inequities. They pertain in large part to macrosocial of health (the health consideration introduced in the AVMSD still has more to do with regulating corporate practices that influence behaviour). Finally, we have looked at the space for HiAP in the EC meta-regulatory landscape, given that HiAP is supposed to be mainstreamed, which means that it is supposed to permeate all EU activities. The examples of Better Regulation and the collegiality principle, which are elements of meta-regulation, reflect the EU constitutional asymmetry.

Each section has provided a glimpse into the difficulties of implementing HiAP and taking up a radically broad understanding of health promotion. Looking at the relationships between the various sections, it is also clear how a minimalist understanding of health promotion as limited to proximal determinants of health sits neatly in the constitutional asymmetry context. Policy areas which have a bearing on macrosocial determinants of health tend to fall within the remit of harder and meta-regulatory governance, where the perceived relevance to health is limited and where the goals pursued are economic in nature (growth, competitiveness, etc.), while proximal, risk-factors-related public health promotion remains governed by 'soft' methods directed at disciplining and responsibilising individuals and corporations. This is illustrative of the EU institutional neoliberal bias. Importantly, and as pointed out elsewhere (Greer, 2014), promoting population health is not the main objective even of EU activities related to health, let alone in activities of other DGs. Promoting health across sectors, based on growing understandings of the complexity and interdependencies that shape public health burdens, would entail considerable priority shifts not only in DG SANTE and in health policies, but across DGs and non-health policies (as well as across EU institutions). As suggested earlier, the fact that member states are reluctant to confer healthcare and health system competencies on the EU does not in any way undermine or cancel the obligation of the EU to enhance and/or promote population health and wellbeing through all its *other* actions. When taking a broad conceptualisation of health promotion, as outlined in the previous chapter, it should become clear that HiAP is not about subsidiarity infringement, but about creating the policy space for prioritising societal health and wellbeing.

The neoliberal institutional structures, in a 'conventional' sense, however, do not tell the whole story of why HiAP fails to be taken up at EU level. This institutional configuration, however powerfully anchored, did not 'happen' out of the blue and does not sustain itself independently, without an underlying cognitive and linguistic system of meaning to support, reinforce and sometimes challenge it. In other words, constitutional asymmetry is unlikely to be the only factor standing in the way of HiAP at EU level. At the same time, the dominant institutional dynamics are not homogeneous, given that HiAP was elevated to the EU agenda in the first place. Limiting the analysis of HiAP at EU level to institutional factors would fail to capture underlying dynamics that shape those factors, and it would run the risk of presenting institutions as immutable, regular entities that operate in a predictable, monolithic fashion. Instead, this book argues for the need to look beyond constitutional asymmetry and the soft/hard governance dichotomy to analyse the power in dominant ideas and representations of health and knowledge, before highlighting the spaces for contestation in the meanings of ideas. Going back to the various elements in Schmidt's DI, the next chapter will take a closer look at the ideational obstacles to HiAP, or what this book refers to as 'background ideational structures'.

References

Ackrill, R., Kay, A., & Morgan, W. (2008). The common agricultural policy and its reform: The problem of reconciling budget and trade concerns. *Canadian Journal of Agricultural Economics, 56*, 393–411.

Azzopardi-Muscat, N., Clemens, T., Stoner, D., & Brand, H. (2015). EU Country Specific Recommendations for health systems in the European Semester process: Trends, discourse and predictors. *Health Policy, 119*(3), 375–383.

Azzopardi-Muscat, N., & Brand, H. (2014). The 'European Semester'—A growing force shaping Health Systems Policy and Reform in the European Union. *European Journal of Public Health, 24*(2), 232.

Bache, I., Bulmer, S., George, S., & Parker, O. (2015). *Politics in the European Union* (4th ed.). Oxford University Press.

Baum, F., Delany-Crowe, T., MacDougall, C., van Eyk, H., Lawless, A., Williams, C., & Marmot , M. (2019). To what extent can the activities of the South Australian Health in All Policies initiative be linked to population health outcomes using a program theory-based evaluation? *BMC Public Health, 19*(88), https://doi.org/10.1186/s12889-019-6408-y

Baum, F., & Fisher, M. (2014). Why behavioural health promotion endures despite its failure to reduce health inequities. *Sociology of Health and Illness, 36*(2), 213–225.

Borrás, S., & Jacobsson, K. (2004). The open method of co-ordination and new governance patterns in the EU. *Journal of European Public Policy, 11*(2), 185–208.
Bruno, I., Jacquot, S., & Mandin, L. (2006). Europeanization through its instrumentation: Benchmarking, mainstreaming and the open method of co-ordination…toolbox or Pandora's box? *Journal of European Public Policy, 13*(4), 519–536.
Carey, G., Malbon, E., Crammond, B., Pescud, M., & Baker, P. (2017). Can the sociology of social problems help us to understand and manage 'lifestyle drift'? *Health Promotion International, 32*(4), 755–761.
Costa, H., Gilmore, A. B., Peeters, S., McKee, M., & Stuckler, D. (2014). Quantifying the influence of the tobacco industry on EU governance: Automated content analysis of the EU Tobacco Products Directive. *Tobacco Control, 23*(6), 473–478.
De la Porte, C., & Nanz, P. (2004). The OMC—A deliberative-democratic mode of governance? The cases of employment and pensions. *Journal of European Public Policy, 11*(2), 267–288.
De la Porte, C., & Pochet, P. (2012). Why and how (still) study the Open Method of Co-ordination (OMC)? *Journal of European Social Policy, 22*(3), 336–349.
Douglas, M. (2015). Beyond 'health': Why don't we tackle the cause of health inequalities? In K. E. Smith, C. Bambra, & S. Hill (Eds.), *Health inequalities—Critical Perspectives* (pp. 109–123). Oxford University Press.
EurActive. (2015, June 3). *Health NGOs walk out of EU alcohol forum*. https://www.euractiv.com/section/health-consumers/news/health-ngos-walk-out-of-eu-alcohol-forum/. Accessed 15 November 2019.
EuroHealthNet. (2018, November). *The European semester 2018 from a health equity perspective*. https://eurohealthnet.eu/sites/eurohealthnet.eu/files/publications/The%20European%20Semester%202018%20from%20a%20health%20equity%20perspective.pdf. Accessed 15 November 2019.
European Commission. (2007, May 30). *A strategy for Europe on nutrition, overweight and obesity related health issues* [White paper]. Brussels. COM(2007) 279 final. https://eur-lex.europa.eu/LexUriServ/LexUriServ.do?uri=COM:2007:0279:FIN:EN:PDF. Accessed 13 November 2019.
European Commission. (2008). *EU framework for national salt initiatives [High Level Group on Nutrition and Physical Activity]*. https://ec.europa.eu/health/ph_determinants/life_style/nutrition/documents/salt_initiative.pdf. Accessed 12 November 2019.
European Commission. (2009, January 15). *Impact assessment guidelines*. SEC (2009) 92. https://ec.europa.eu/smart-regulation/impact/commission_guidelines/docs/iag_2009_en.pdf. Accessed 15 July 2019.

European Commission. (2011). *EU Framework for National Initiatives on Selected Nutrients* [High Level Group on Nutrition and Physical Activity]. https://ec.europa.eu/health/sites/health/files/nutrition_physical_activity/docs/euframework_national_nutrients_en.pdf. Accessed 12 November 2019.

European Commission. (2012). *Annex 1: Saturated Fat. EU framework for national initiatives on selected nutrients*. [High Level Group on Nutrition and Physical Activity]. https://ec.europa.eu/health//sites/health/files/nutrition_physical_activity/docs/satured_fat_eufnisn_en.pdf. Accessed 12 November 2019.

European Commission. (2014a). *The working methods of the European Commission 2014–2019* [Communication from the President to the Commission]. https://ec.europa.eu/info/sites/info/files/the_working_methods_of_the_european_commission_2014-2019_november2014_en.pdf. Accessed 12 November 2019.

European Commission. (2014b, April 4). *Communication from the Commission on effective, accessible and resilient health systems*. Brussels. COM(2014) 215 final. https://ec.europa.eu/health//sites/health/files/systems_performance_assessment/docs/com2014_215_final_en.pdf. Accessed 12 November 2019.

European Commission. (2015a, May 19). *Better regulation for better results—An EU agenda* [Communication from the Commission to the European Parliament, the European Economic and Social Committee and the Committee of the Regions] Strasbourg. https://eur-lex.europa.eu/legal-content/EN/TXT/PDF/?uri=CELEX:52015DC0215&from=EN. Accessed 12 November 2019.

European Commission. (2015b). *Annex 2: Added sugars. EU framework for national initiatives on selected nutrients* [High Level Group on Nutrition and Physical Activity]. https://ec.europa.eu/health//sites/health/files/nutrition_physical_activity/docs/added_sugars_en.pdf. Accessed 12 November 2019.

European Commission. (2015c, July 6–September 30). *Synopsis report of the Public consultation on Directive 2010/13/EU on Audiovisual Media Services (AVMSD)—A media framework for the 21st century*. PDF download available from: https://ec.europa.eu/digital-single-market/en/news/report-public-consultation-review-audiovisual-media-services-directive-avmsd. Accessed 12 November 2019.

European Commission. (2015d). *Ex-post Evaluation of the Health Programme (2008–2013)*. Final Report. https://ec.europa.eu/health/sites/health/files/programme/docs/ex-post_ev-hp-2008-13_final-report.pdf. Accessed 12 November 2019.

European Commission. (2016a, May). *Monitoring the activities of the EU Platform for Action on Diet, Physical Activity and Health: Annual Report 2016* [Written by ICF Consulting Services Ltd]. https://www.icsspe.org/system/files/European%20Commission%20-%20Monitoring%20the%20activities%20of%20the%20EU%20Platform%20for%20Action%20on%20Diet%2C%20Physical%20Activity%20and%20Health%202016.pdf. Accessed 12 November 2019.

European Commission. (2016b). Proposal for a Directive of the European Parliament and of the Council amending Directive 2010/13/EU on the coordination of certain provisions laid down by law, regulation or administration action in Member States concerning the provision of audiovisual media services in view of changing market realities. Brussels, 25 May. COM(2016) 287 final, 2016/0151 (COD). https://eur-lex.europa.eu/legal-content/EN/TXT/PDF/?uri=CELEX:52016PC0287&from=GA. Accessed 12 November 2019.

European Commission. (2016c, January 15). *Mapping of the use of European structural and investment funds in health in the 2007–2013 and 2014–2020 programming periods*. https://www.esifforhealth.eu/pdf/Mapping_Report_Final.pdf. Accessed 12 November 2019.

European Commission. (2016d). *European Semester Thematic Factsheet: Sustainability of Public Finances*. https://ec.europa.eu/info/sites/info/files/european-semester_thematic-factsheet_public-finance-sustainability_en_0.pdf. Accessed 18 March 2019.

European Commission. (2017a). *Better regulation 'toolbox'*. https://ec.europa.eu/info/sites/info/files/better-regulation-toolbox_2.pdf. Accessed 12 November 2019.

European Commission. (2017b, July 7). *Better regulation guidelines* [Commission Staff Working Document]. Brussels. SWD (2017) 350. https://ec.europa.eu/info/sites/info/files/better-regulation-guidelines.pdf. Accessed 12 November 2019.

European Commission. (2017c). *Modernising & simplifying the CAP: Socio-economic challenges facing agriculture and rural areas*. https://ec.europa.eu/agriculture/sites/agriculture/files/consultations/cap-modernising/soc_background_final_en.pdf. Accessed 12 November 2019.

European Commission. (2017d). *European semester thematic factsheet: Health systems*. https://ec.europa.eu/info/sites/info/files/file_import/european-semester_thematic-factsheet_health-systems_en_0.pdf. Accessed 18 March 2019.

European Commission. (2017e, December 20). *Strategic Plan 2016–2020: DG health & food safety*. https://ec.europa.eu/info/sites/info/files/strategic-plan-2016-2020-dg-sante_en_0.pdf. Accessed 28 March 2019.

European Commission. (2018a, February 23). *Platform members*. https://ec.europa.eu/health/sites/health/files/nutrition_physical_activity/docs/platform_members_en.pdf. Accessed 12 November 2019.

European Commission. (2018b, June). *EU budget: The CAP after 2020: Modernising & Simplifying the Common Agricultural Policy*. https://ec.europa.eu/commission/sites/beta-political/files/budget-may2018-modernising-cap_en.pdf. Accessed 13 November 2019.

European Commission. (2018c, June 1). Proposal for a Regulation of the European Parliament and of the Council establishing rules on support for strategic plans to be drawn up by Member States under the Common agricultural policy (CAP Strategic Plans) [...] Brussels. COM(2018) 392 final. 2018/0216 (COD). https://eur-lex.europa.eu/resource.html?uri=cellar:aa85fa9a-65a0-11e8-ab9c-01aa75ed71a1.0003.02/DOC_1&format=PDF. Accessed 12 November 2019.

European Commission. (2018d, June 1). Proposal for a Regulation of the European Parliament and of the Council on the financing, management and monitoring of the common agricultural policy and repealing Regulation (EU) No 1306/2013. Brussels. COM (2018) 393 final. 2018/0217 (COD). https://eur-lex.europa.eu/resource.html?uri=cellar:6cb59a1e-6580-11e8-ab9c-01aa75ed71a1.0003.03/DOC_1&format=PDF. Accessed 12 November 2019.

European Commission. (2018e, June 1). Annexes to the proposal for a regulation of the European Parliament and of the Council establishing rules on support for strategic plans to be drawn up by Member States under the Common Agricultural Policy (CAP strategic plans) Brussels. COM(2018) 392 final ANNEXES 1 to 12. https://eur-lex.europa.eu/resource.html?uri=cellar:aa85fa9a-65a0-11e8-ab9c-01aa75ed71a1.0003.02/DOC_2&format=PDF. Accessed 12 November 2019.

European Commission. (2019a). The post-2020 Common Agricultural Policy: Environmental benefits and simplification. https://ec.europa.eu/info/sites/info/files/food-farming-fisheries/key_policies/documents/cap-post-2020-environ-benefits-simplification_en.pdf. Accessed 23 May 2019.

European Commission. (2019b). *ESI Funds for Health: Investing for a healthy and inclusive EU. Final Report*. http://www.esifundsforhealth.eu/sites/default/files/2019-03/Final%20Report%20ESI%20Funds%20for%20Health_2.pdf. Accessed 12 November 2019.

European Commission. (2020a). A Farm to Fork Strategy for a fair, healthy and environmentally-friendly food system. COM(2020) 381 final. https://eur-lex.europa.eu/resource.html?uri=cellar:ea0f9f73-9ab2-11ea-9d2d-01aa75ed71a1.0001.02/DOC_1&format=PDF. Accessed 17 September 2021.

European Commission. (2020b). EU Biodiversity Strategy for 2030 Bringing nature back into our lives. COM(2020) 380 final. https://eur-lex.europa.

eu/resource.html?uri=cellar:a3c806a6-9ab3-11ea-9d2d-01aa75ed71a1.0001.02/DOC_1&format=PDF. Accessed 17 September 2021.

European Commission. (2020c). Working with Parliament and Council to make the CAP reform fit for the European Green Deal. Factsheet. https://ec.europa.eu/info/sites/default/files/food-farming-fisheries/key_policies/documents/factsheet-cap-reform-to-fit-european-green-deal_en.pdf. Accessed 17 September 2021.

European Commission. (n.d.a). *EU Platform for action on diet, physical activity and health* [Website]. https://ec.europa.eu/health/nutrition_physical_activity/platform_en. Accessed 21 December 2016.

European Commission. (n.d.b). *High level group on nutrition and physical activity* [Website]. https://ec.europa.eu/health/nutrition_physical_activity/high_level_group_en. Accessed 8 October 2019.

European Commission. (n.d.c). *The common agricultural policy at a glance* [Website]. https://ec.europa.eu/info/food-farming-fisheries/key-policies/common-agricultural-policy/cap-glance_en. Accessed 12 November 2019.

European Heart Network, The European Consumer Organisation, European Public Health Alliance, World Obesity, COFACE Families Europe, et al. (2019a, July 3). *Civil Society Organisations leave the EU platform for diet, physical activity and health* [Open Letter]. https://epha.org/wp-content/uploads/2019/07/joint-statement-leaving-eu-diet-and-physical-activity-platform-july2019.pdf. Accessed 15 November 2019.

European Heart Network, The European Consumer Organisation, European Public Health Alliance, World Obesity, COFACE Families Europe, et al. (2019b). Joint letter by consumer groups and public health organisations on the need for a review of the objectives and functioning of the EU Platform on Diet, Physical Activity and Health. https://epha.org/wp-content/uploads/2019/07/joint-letter-i-diet-and-physical-activity-platform-04-2019.pdf. Accessed 15 November 2019.

European Parliament. (2017). REPORT on the proposal for a directive of the European Parliament and of the Council amending Directive 2010/13/EU on the coordination of certain provisions laid down by law, regulation or administrative action in Member States concerning the provision of audiovisual media services in view of changing market realities (COM(2016)0287 – C8-0193/2016 – 2016/0151(COD)). http://www.europarl.europa.eu/doceo/document/A-8-2017-0192_EN.pdf. Accessed 12 November 2019.

European Parliament. (2019, January 25). *The audiovisual media services directive* (6th ed.) [Briefing EU Legislation in Progress]. http://www.europarl.europa.eu/RegData/etudes/BRIE/2016/583859/EPRS_BRI%282016%29583859_EN.pdf. Accessed 12 November 2019.

European Public Health Alliance. (2016a). *3 Steps towards healthier marketing—Improve the AVMDS*. https://epha.org/3-steps-towards-healthier-marketing-improve-the-avmsd/. Accessed 13 November 2019.
European Public Health Alliance. (2016b). *AVMSD: Once in a Decade Opportunity to protect children from unhealthy marketing* [Press release]. https://epha.org/press-release-avmsd-once-in-a-decade-opportunity-to-protect-children-from-unhealthy-marketing/. Accessed 13 November 2019.
European Public Health Alliance. (2016c). *A CAP for healthy living: Mainstreaming health into the EU common agricultural policy* [Report]. https://epha.org/wp-content/uploads/2016/03/A-CAP-for-Healthy-Living_EPHA_2016.pdf. Accessed 13 November 2019.
European Public Health Alliance. (2017). *Ministerial Action needed to improve AVMSD* [Open Letter]. https://epha.org/open-letter-i-ministerial-action-needed-to-improve-avmsd/. Accessed 13 November 2019.
European Public Health Alliance. (2018). *The New CAP: Great promise of give-away?* [Notes on leaked proposal]. https://epha.org/the-new-cap-great-promise-or-give-away-notes-on-the-leaked-proposal/. Accessed 13 November 2019.
European Union. (2018). Directive (EU) 2018/1808 of the European Parliament and of the Council amending Directive 2010/13/EU on the coordination of certain provisions laid down by law, regulation or administrative action in Member States concerning the provision of audiovisual media services (Audiovisual Media Services Directive) in view of changing market realities. *Official Journal of the European Union*. https://eur-lex.europa.eu/legal-content/EN/TXT/PDF/?uri=CELEX:32018L1808&qid=1550491395985&from=en. Accessed 12 November 2019.
Garde, A., Jeffery, B., & Rigby, N. (2017). Implementing the WHO recommendations whilst avoiding real, perceived or potential conflicts of interest. *European Journal of Risk Regulation, 8*(2), 237–250.
Garriga, E., & Melé, D. (2004). Corporate social responsibility theories: Mapping the territory. *Journal of Business Ethics, 53*, 51–71.
Garzon, I. (2006). *Reforming the common agricultural policy: History of a paradigm change*. Palgrave Macmillan.
Greer, S. L. (2014). Three faces of European Union Health Policy: Policy, markets, and austerity. *Policy and Society, 33*(1), 13–24.
Herrick, C. (2009). Shifting blame/selling health: Corporate social responsibility in the age of obesity. *Sociology of Health and Illness, 31*(1), 51–65.
Kemm, J. (2006). Health impact assessment and Health in All Policies. In T. Ståhl, M. Wismar, E. Ollila, Lahtinen, E., & Leppo, K. (Eds.), *Health in All Policies: Prospect and potentials* (pp. 189–208). Ministry of Social Affairs and Health, Finland.

Kohler-Koch, B., & Finke, B. (2007). The institutional shaping of EU-Society relations: A contribution to democracy via participation? *Journal of Civil Society, 3*(3), 205–221.

Koivusalo, M. (2010). The state of Health in All Policies (HiAP) in the European Union: Potential and pitfalls. *Journal of Epidemiology and Community Health, 64*(6), 500–503.

Kröger, S. (2007). The end of democracy as we know it? The legitimacy deficits of bureaucratic social policy governance. *Journal of European Integration, 29*(5), 565–582.

Merkel, B. (2010). *Health in All Policies 2010—Dr. Bernard Merkel* [Video uploaded on Vimeo]. *SA Health Conference, Government of South Australia.* https://vimeo.com/13389841. Accessed 13 November 2019.

Moodie, R., Stuckler, D., Monteiro, C., Sheron, N., Neal, B., Thamarangsi, T., Lincoln, P., Casswell, S., & Lancet NCD Action Group. (2013). Profits and pandemics: Prevention of harmful effects of tobacco, alcohol, and ultra-processed food and drink industries. *The Lancet, 381*(9867), 670–679.

Parker, O. (2008). Challenging 'new constitutionalism' in the EU: French resistance, 'Social Europe' and 'Soft' governance. *New Political Economy, 13*(4), 397–417.

Parkhurst, J. (2017). *The politics of evidence: From evidence-based policy to the good governance of evidence*. Routledge.

Pe'er, G., Zinngrebe, Y., Moreira, F., Sirami, C., Schindler, S., Müller, R., Bontzorlos, V., Clough, D., Bezák, P., Bonn, A., Hansjürgens, B., Lomba, A., Möckel, S., Passoni, G., Schleyer, C., Schmidt, J., & Lakner, S. (2019). A greener path for the EU Common Agricultural Policy. *Science, 365*(6452), 449–451.

Peeters, S., Costa, H., Stuckler, D., McKee, M., & Gilmore, A. B. (2016). The revision of the 2014 European tobacco products directive: An analysis of the tobacco industry's attempt to 'break the health silo.' *Tobacco Control, 25*(1), 108–117.

Popay, J., Whitehead, M., & Hunter, D. (2010). Editorial: Injustice is killing people on a large scale—But what is to be done about it? *Journal of Public Health, 32*(2), 148–149.

Powell, K., Thurston, M., & Bloyce, D. (2017). Theorising lifestyle drift in health promotion: Explaining community and voluntary sector engagement practices in disadvantaged areas. *Critical Public Health, 27*(5), 554–565.

Radulova, E. (2007). The OMC: An opaque method of consideration of deliberative governance in action? *Journal of European Integration, 29*(3), 363–380.

Roederer-Rynning, C., & Matthews, A. (2019). What common agricultural policy after Brexit? *Politics and Governance, 7*(3), 40–50.

Ronit, K., & Jensen, J. D. (2014). Obesity and industry self-regulation of food and beverage marketing: A literature review. *European Journal of Clinical Nutrition, 68*(7), 753–759.

Shore, C. (2011). 'European Governance' or governmentality? The European Commission and the future of democratic government. *European Law Journal, 17*(3), 287–303.

Smismans, S. (2008). New modes of governance and the participatory myth. *West European Politics, 31*(5), 874–895.

Smith, K. E. (2013). *Beyond evidence-based policy in public health: The interplay of ideas*. Palgrave Macmillan.

Smith, K. E., Fooks, G., Collin, J., Weishaar, H., Mandal, S., & Gilmore, A. B. (2010a). "Working the system"—British American Tobacco's Influence on the European Union Treaty and its implications for policy: An analysis of internal tobacco industry documents. *PLoS Medicine, 7*(1). https://doi.org/10.1371/journal.pmed.1000202

Smith, K. E., Fooks, G., Collin, J., Weishaar, H., & Gilmore, A. B. (2010). Is the increasing policy use of Impact Assessment in European likely to undermine efforts to achieve healthy public policy? *Journal of Epidemiology and Community Health, 64*(6), 478–487.

Smith, K. E., Fooks, G., Gilmore, A. B., Collin, J., & Weishaar, H. (2015). Corporate coalitions and policymaking in the European Union: How and why British American Tobacco promoted 'Better Regulation.' *Journal of Health Politics, Policy and Law, 40*(2), 325–372.

Smith, K. E., Gilmore, A. B., Fooks, G., Collin, J., & Weishaar, H. (2009). Tobacco industry attempts to undermine Article 5.3 and the 'good governance' trap. *Tobacco Control, 18*(6), 509–511.

Thornley, L., Signal, L., & Thomson, G. (2010). Does industry regulation of food advertising protect child rights? *Critical Public Health, 20*(1), 25–33.

Walls, H. L., Cornelsen, L., Lock, K., & Smith, R. D. (2016). How much priority is given to nutrition and health in the EU Common Agricultural Policy? *Food Policy, 59*, 12–23.

Wilkinson, R. G., & Pickett, K. (2010). *The spirit level: Why equality is better for everyone* (2nd ed.). Penguin Books.

Williams, O., & Fullagar, S. (2019). Lifestyle drift and the phenomenon of 'citizen shift' in contemporary UK health policy. *Sociology of Health and Illness, 41*(1), 20–35.

Zeitlin, J., & Vanhercke, B. (2014, December). *Socializing the European semester? Economic governance and social policy coordination in Europe 2020*. Swedish Institute for European Policy Studies [Report no. 7].

CHAPTER 6

Going Deeper: Is It About More Than Institutions?

If the institutional imbalances explored earlier were redressed, would HiAP be automatically better implemented? I suggest that the obstacles to meaningfully considering macrosocial determinants of health are about more than the purely institutional structures. To understand the ideational barriers to HiAP, we need to look at established worldviews and shared understandings of meanings prevailing in the EU. First, we need to look at 'health' itself. Health and health promotion can be understood in different ways, with different underlying norms and values. This chapter explores how, in the EU, health tends to be seen through an economic lens that interacts with security and biomedical paradigms. The chapter then explores why these ways of conceptualising health do not fit well with a kind of HiAP that would address macrosocial determinants of health and health inequities, and how that represents an ideational barrier to HiAP in the EU. Second, we need to look at how the European Commission defines what represents legitimate and useable evidence, and what implications this has for HiAP. I argue that the complexity and normativity of HiAP do not fit into a dominant knowledge paradigm, where evidence is expected to be apolitical and measurable.

The previous chapter told part of the story of why HiAP struggles to be taken up due constraining institutional structures. However, the institutional architecture is not the only dimension that reflects a

C. Godziewski, *The Politics of Health Promotion*, Palgrave Studies in Science, Knowledge and Policy, https://doi.org/10.1007/978-3-030-97870-9_6

neoliberal rationality. Furthermore, the institutional architecture does not sustain itself on its own, independently of ideational and discursive dynamics. Going beyond 'conventional' institutionalism means rejecting the assumption that, if the soft governance areas were stronger and able to counterbalance the weight of hard governance, then little would stand in the way of HiAP. Or, more generally, that little would stand in the way of a less neoliberal, more social EU. Rather, one also needs to consider underlying systems of meanings, or to put it in DI terms, the 'background ideational structures', in order to better capture how neoliberalism is reproduced ideationally, through frames, their embeddedness in paradigms, and how paradigms are shaped by neoliberal rationality.

The analysis in this chapter suggests that a neoliberal rationality is reflected in paradigms of health and of knowledge, as well as in the framings of NCDs and evidence which they induce. Note that paradigms should not be thought of as somehow *independent* of 'conventional' institutional dynamics seen previously. Quite the opposite: the concept of constitutional asymmetry explored earlier, for example, is closely related to the economic paradigm of health. Arguably, one could think of these two concepts as two manifestations of neoliberal rationality which reinforce each other: constitutional asymmetry being the institutional manifestation, and the economic paradigm of health as the ideational one. I do not argue, then, that the ideational and the institutional sides of the coin are somehow separate. Rather, this chapter explores ways in which the multiple different paradigms and frames reproduce neoliberal rationality while being mobilised *in spaces other than the constitutional asymmetry*. In turn, this chapter is concerned with Schmidt's second element of DI, the background ideational structures. To get a better sense of what happens to HiAP at the EU, it is necessary to look beyond the soft/hard governance divide, aligned with a conceptualisation of power in binary terms. Here we look at power *in* ideas, power as present in language and reproduced through knowledge production and meaning-making. This suggests a simultaneously more pervasive presence of neoliberal rationality, but also a less rigid, less inevitable one.

This chapter uses discourse analysis to explore the interactions between paradigms and frames and how neoliberalism permeates and is reinforced through them. Starting with briefly presenting various paradigms of health that have been argued to fit neatly with neoliberal rationality, it zooms into and focuses on the economic paradigm of health and how it manifests at the EU level. We will explore recurrent themes and ideational pathways through which health is repeatedly thought of in relation to economic growth and see how the economic paradigm of health dominates in the EU in relation to NCDs and health promotion. The following part of the chapter looks at how the economic paradigm of health, in conjunction and overlapping with the security and the biomedical paradigms of health, shapes the framing of NCDs. The implications of these frames and paradigms for HiAP, and their rootedness in a 'neoliberal deep core', are then reflected upon. The second half of the chapter identifies and describes the positivist, hypothetico-deductive knowledge paradigm as dominant in the EU context. This is visible through the theme of 'evidence', and what is considered usable and legitimate evidence. Here, the analysis puts in relation frames of evidence, with the positivist paradigm of knowledge, and the neoliberal 'deep core' which underpins that paradigm.

Dominant health and knowledge paradigms, and their normative underpinning, are mutually reinforcing. Dominant paradigms and frames have important implications in terms of scope to take up HiAP. This is particularly the case in relation to the normativity and complexity of HiAP. Figure 6.1 provides an overview of this chapter's rationale, and how its argument is structured. Ultimately, this chapter makes the point that, in the EU context, HiAP is not only undermined by a prevailing (neoliberal) constitutional asymmetry, but also by a neoliberal ideational asymmetry. While both are co-constitutive and therefore related, that the latter is *more* than a simple consequence of the former.

6.1 The Economic Paradigm of Health

The economic paradigm of health tends to value action and investment in public health because of its return on investment and the profitability of this market: health is worth investing in, because for each euro invested, the return is much higher. Investing in health is also a good opportunity to foster economic growth. This is a common way of thinking about health governance and policy. It monetises the value of promoting health in a bid to raise public health higher on the agenda priorities. This is a very common—arguably the dominant—paradigm of health visible in EU publications. The logic of the economic paradigm of health in the context of NCDs is that ill-health is expensive, and that it is therefore preferable to invest in health promotion than to pay the cost of curative healthcare and lost productivity (European Commission, 2013a, pp. 4–5; 2014a, p. 2; 2017d). In addition, the economic paradigm of health

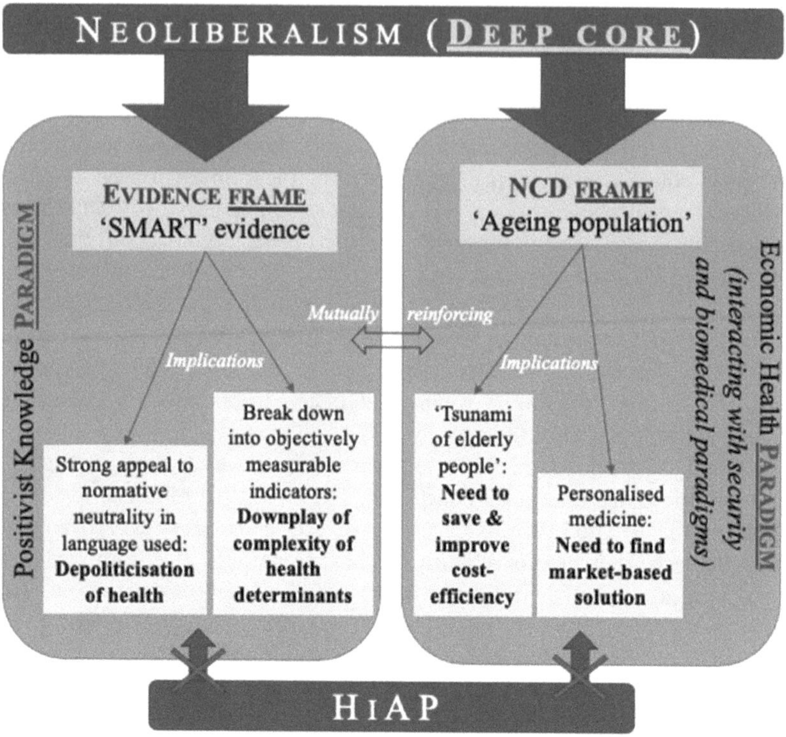

Fig. 6.1 Chapter overview: exploring EU background ideational structures

conceptualises health as a vibrant economic field with a lot of innovative potential which, when harnessed, can bring about economic growth (European Commission, 2014a, p. 3; 2017d; 2017h). One important disclaimer is that this paradigm is by no means specific to the EU. Indeed, the economic paradigm of health has been widespread at global, international and national levels elsewhere, for a while now (see, e.g., Jamison et al., 2016; OECD, 2010; Sachs, 2001).

Aligned with that paradigm, numerous EC public health documents (e.g. European Commission, 2017d; 2017g) start with an acknowledgement that health is a desirable goal in and of itself and a human right, only to then emphasise the financial cost of ill-health, the loss of productivity that results from ill-health, and the amount of money and economic growth that could be generated if the population was healthier. Economic language seems to be the most 'serious' and legitimate explanation, and the human rights language does not carry the same weight and is merely cited *en passant*. In a way reminiscent of the 'lifestyle drift', there tends to be an 'economic drift' when talking about the importance of health in the EU space: it starts off with recognising the importance of health on its own right, only to drift into focusing on the impacts on the economy (see European Commission, 2014a; 2017a, p. 10; 2019a, p. 17). Here is an example of this discursive tendency:

> Besides being a value in itself, health is also a precondition for economic prosperity, as recognised in the Commission staff working document 'Investing in health', which is part of the Social Investment Package. People's health influences economic outcomes in terms of productivity, labour supply, human capital and public spending. (European Commission, 2014a, p. 3)

The ubiquity of the economic paradigm of health does not mean that all individuals working in relevant fields value it more than rights-based justifications for health. One interviewee in particular insisted that, far from being a preference, adopting the language of health as a means for economic growth is something inevitable, a necessity if health is to be heard by other policy areas.[1]

The link between health and economic growth is well researched, and even some critical public health practitioners have stressed the power and usefulness of highlighting and using this link to advance the public health cause.[2] They argue that it is not something public health experts should reject or downplay, as long as they remain acutely aware of the risk of co-option, and the necessity of seeing the economic argument as a tool to achieve health and wellbeing, rather than the other way around. In that vein, the aim of this chapter section is not to critique the point that good health contributes to economic prosperity. Similarly, economic prosperity matters and is an important condition for people to live fulfilling and emancipated lives. The point of critique, however, is the dominance of the economic paradigm of health over the reasoning that health should genuinely be seen as a goal in itself, not only in the health sector, but in

[1] Source: interviewee 8.

[2] Source: interviewees 31 and 27.

other policy areas as well (HiAP). As will be detailed below, and as already argued by others (Baum & Fisher, 2014; Smith, 2013), the economic paradigm of health is unlikely to lead to an approach to health which adequately prioritises health equity. As such, it is an impediment to HiAP and represents a manifestation of neoliberal rationality in public health policy, whereby economic thinking intrudes into all areas of life. The economic paradigm of health presents two main faces: on the one hand, health promotion and public health is seen in terms of return on investment, as a way to avoid costs related to ill-health. At the same time, health is seen as a market ripe for profit-making. The two faces of the economic paradigm are often present together.

Ill-Health as a Financial Burden to Avoid

The first face—health promotion and disease prevention as a necessary investment to prevent healthcare costs spiralling out of control—is exemplified in the quote below:

> 80% of healthcare cost are going on chronic diseases. And therefore, the member states are very anxious to make sure that the drivers of this epidemic are slowed down. And therefore, we need to step up prevention and promotion as much as possible. Because otherwise the health systems are not sustainable. (Quoted from interviewee 28)

Investing in health is then seen first and foremost as a way to minimise a financial burden, rather than for the sake of creating a healthy, thriving and fair society. This does not mean that the two are necessarily mutually exclusive, and it does not question policymakers genuine concern about public health. However, the logic of priority matters enormously, as while both orders of priority recognise that health leads to economic prosperity, both are fundamentally differing in terms of underlying values and worldviews: instead of working towards creating health and wellbeing for its own sake and taking on a paradigmatically 'salutogenic' approach to health promotion, thinking of health promotion as primarily a way to cut healthcare costs reflects a 'pathogenic' approach to health, focused on risk factors to minimise, rather than a public good to maximise. The absence of willingness to adopt a more salutogenic approach to thinking about health, health promotion and NCDs can be seen in this quote from an MEP:

> Prevention for example, I proposed to appoint a Commissioner for prevention. Because the money we allocate for health disappears in the hospitals more or less. But prevention means to work with healthy people and prevention is still not considered as an economic category but when you land in the hospital then you become an economic category. (Quoted from interviewee 24)[3]

What this quote suggests, is that the dominant way to think about health is in terms of economic cost, which rises when people are ill and need to use the health system. This reflects a pathogenic approach to health, which focuses on ill-health treatment—and prevention for the sake of cost-saving—rather than focusing on health and wellbeing generation. What is lacking, is a vision for creating a healthy, wellbeing society. As expressed in the quote above, EU added value is perceived as justified when it comes to creating more cost-effective, modern health systems ready to cope with the 'economic category' of (elderly) chronically sick people, but not when it comes to imagining and creating a world in which fewer people would be chronically sick. In that area, the scope for what is conceivable for the EU to do in terms of health promotion is reduced to merely fostering knowledge and best practice exchange among member states. Note, however, that the quote of the MEP itself shows that actors within the institutions can be critical of their institutions, and points to the existence of discursive spaces of agency.[4]

Health as a Lucrative Market

The other face of the economic paradigm of health is to argue that the health sector represents a great sector for producing wealth. Here, the idea is that health is a large sector of the economy and has a lot of potential for innovation and wealth creation on the global market. This rationale can be found in numerous EU documents (see DG SANTE Strategic Plan for 2016–2020, but also European Commission documents in relation to the 'personalised medicine' priority: European Commission, 2017h, European Commission, n.d.e). By and large, most of the EU health-related funded research concerns pharmaceutical and medical device innovation, as well as innovations for digital solutions, and a

[3] The same idea was suggested by interviewees 17, 18 and 19.

[4] That MEP was involved in the organisation of the Post-Growth conference.

general favouring of projects developing personalised medicine (European Commission, 2015b, 2017e, 2019b).[5] The rationale of health as a profit-making market carries the obvious risk that priorities will be guided not by what has the greatest societal value, but what will lead to profit through marketing treatments or devices which might be useful to some people—especially wealthier people—but would do little to promote health on a societal level and reduce inequities.

This face of the economic paradigm of health is visible, for example, in the creation of the first subgroup within the Steering Group for health promotion, disease prevention and management of NCDs (SGPP) (European Commission, 2018a, 2018b). The purpose of the SGPP is to 'provide strategic advice to the Commission and a forum for consultation among member states on the strategic planning of health promotion as well as prevention and management of non-communicable diseases' (European Commission, 2016b, p. 1). The mandate of the SGPP is unequivocally about gathering knowledge and discussing broad strategies for health promotion and disease prevention in particular in relation to NCDs. Yet the EC decided to create a time-bound, topic-specific subgroup on proton therapy within the SGPP (European Commission, 2018a, p. 5; 2018b). Proton therapy is a high-tech innovative cancer treatment which 'can be effective in particular for highly specialised pathologies such as some eye, brain and skull cancers' (European Commission, 2018b, p. 1). The creation of this subgroup was requested by the European Investment Bank (EIB), which had been approached with proton therapy financing requests (p. 1). Notwithstanding the importance of the availability of treatment for the patients concerned, the matter of the subgroup has no relevance whatsoever to public health promotion. The existence of this subgroup was not mentioned by any of the interviewees talking about the SGPP, and it is unlikely that health policymakers would attempt to present it as public health promotion. But this example illustrates the power of the notion of health as an innovation market leading to resource allocation towards profitable sectors, rather

[5] Exceptions include: PHC 4—2015: Health promotion and disease prevention: improved inter-sector cooperation for environment and health-based interventions (European Commission, 2015b, p. 10), PHC 31—2014: Foresight for health policy development and regulation (European Commission, 2015b, p. 46) and SC1-PM-07-2017: Promoting mental health and well-being in the young (European Commission, 2017e, p. 18).

than focusing on creating more equal and healthy societies. This is not to say that all innovations in health exacerbate inequities, but again, it is about relative weight attributed and prioritisation rationales that the paradigm induces. It is also not to suggest that health promotion in and of itself is incompatible with profit-making: a neoliberal interpretation of health promotion has indeed led to the proliferation of a profitable lifestyle-related market, especially in dieting and exercising (Ayo, 2012), or more recently the commodification of meditation and mindfulness (see part two in Purser et al., 2016). However, the point made in this particular example is that the SGPP was (in part) 'hijacked', and redirected towards researching high-tech specialised medical innovation, even though the group's stated aim is about developing broad strategies for NCD-related health promotion. Since its establishment, the SGPP is developing and working on a variety of topics, including mental health, cancer, nutrition and physical activity and rare diseases.

The co-existence of the two faces of the economic paradigm of health is paradoxical because, while they are compatible in the short-term view of improving cost-efficiency, in the long term it leads to a tension: the profit-making potential of the health sector depends on people getting sick or remaining at risk of getting sick. Of course, people will always be at risk of developing a disease no matter how wellbeing-oriented our societies become. Nevertheless, at its core and in the long term, the market-creating logic of health is conflicting with the need to reduce the financial burden of disease: the aim resulting from these two logics is not to foster a healthier society and fundamentally decrease the number of sick people, but to expand the market to deal with this burden in a cost-effective, or even better, in a profitable way.

The next section looks at how, in interaction with elements of other health paradigms, the economic paradigm of health underpins the dominant framing of NCDs, and how this does not represent an adequate ideational ground to implement HiAP.

6.2 'Ageing Population' Framing of NCDS

One common depiction of NCDs and health promotion tends to portray the burden of NCDs, also often referred to as 'chronic diseases',[6,7] in direct relation to the fact that we live in an ageing society (European Commission, 2000, 2013a; European Union, 2014). The mention of ageing society is present as a justification for action on NCDs and determinants of health, given the threat it will represent in terms of the financial sustainability of health systems. The main health challenge faced by member states that the third Health Programme (HP) identified was the 'demographic context, threatening the sustainability of health systems' (European Commission, 2014c, p. 1). '[B]etter levels of health across all population groups are critical in the context of an ageing EU population to contribute to the sustainability of social protection systems' (European Commission, 2009, p. 5). Another typical example would be:

> In the context of an ageing society, well-directed investments to promote health and prevent diseases can increase the number of 'healthy life years' and thus enable the elderly to enjoy a healthy and active life as they get older. Chronic diseases are responsible for over 80 % of premature mortality in the Union. (European Union, 2014, p. 86/3)

Mentions of 'inequalities' nowadays also often accompany opening statements on NCDs.[8] The rationale of DG SANTE's 2014–2020 public health strategy is based on the identification of various challenges, the first one being: an 'increasingly challenging demographic context threating the sustainability of health systems', along with the increase in prevalence of chronic diseases, as well as the rising inequalities between and within member states (European Commission, 2014b, 2014c). The importance of ageing is very much emphasised and presented as a natural, obvious causal factor for the rise of NCDs. The 'ESIF for Health' report, for example, defines 'health promotion and healthy ageing' as

[6] 'Chronic diseases' refers to the usual NCD (cancer, cardiovascular diseases, diabetes, chronic pulmonary diseases) as well as neurological mental diseases and other diseases like arthritis and allergy-induced respiratory diseases.

[7] https://ec.europa.eu/research/health/index.cfm?pg=area&areaname=chronic.

[8] The way in which the inequality aspect is interpreted and the implications of its interpretation does not invalidate the argument made in this section and will be addressed in section 5.2.2.2, p. 169.

a single thematic category (European Commission, 2019a). Indeed, the EU population is getting older, and with this demographic change, the number of people with NCDs is also growing. This makes sense, given that NCDs such as cancer, cardiovascular diseases and type II diabetes predominantly affect middle-aged and elderly parts of the population compared to young population groups. The point of this section is not to claim that rising NCD prevalence has nothing to do with ageing. Rather, it is about digging deeper into the implications of this framing, exploring how it relates to the economic (and other) paradigms of health, and what is left unacknowledged by this framing. The paragraphs below will elaborate the critique of the framing of NCDs as a (inevitable) result of an ageing population. They show how this framing—like any framing—is not neutral. Rather, it is the product of health paradigms underpinned by neoliberal rationality.

Economic and Security Paradigms: A Tsunami of Elderly People as the Problem

The NCD 'ageing population' frame is fuelled by (and reinforces) the first face of the economic paradigm of health pertaining to ill-health as a financial burden to avoid. Here, the ageing population, with its propensity to develop NCDs, is portrayed as an unavoidable threat to the financial sustainability of the healthcare system (as well as, in combination with low birth rates, the pensions system). 'European population is ageing and more exposed to multiple chronic diseases. This leads to higher demand for healthcare and increasing fiscal pressure' (European Commission, 2017c, p. 1). Given that the process of the ageing population in itself is desirable, the accent is put on how to cope with this imminent threat to healthcare system sustainability. This 'threat' logic resonates with the security paradigm of health (see Elbe, 2006). The security paradigm of health is built on a 'threat-defence' logic and tends to be used mostly in relation to infectious disease control and threats of pandemics or biological warfare (McInnes, 2015). Public and global health issues that receive the most attention have been mostly infectious diseases, likely because they fit best with a traditional conceptualisation of security (Benson & Glasgow, 2015). Yet even beyond pandemic and biological warfare, global health is increasingly conceptualised as a security issue. In the context of NCDs, the security paradigm which emphasises the notion of 'threat', 'risk' and 'crisis', and which is more likely to captivate the attention of policymakers, relates to the strain caused by NCD patients on social services: the image is that of a wave of chronically sick, elderly people which will cause the health system to break down if costs are not saved. The EC talks about 'future-proofing health systems'[9] (European Commission, 2019a, p. 31):

> Population ageing, technological change and growing citizen expectations are placing greater pressure on Member State health budgets. Action will be necessary to ensure the long-term fiscal sustainability of healthcare systems. (European Commission, 2019a, p. 31)

The focus then subtly changes from NCDs themselves to health system sustainability as a matter of economic security. The 'pragmatic' goal is not so much to create a society in which fewer people would develop NCDs, but to improve cost-effectiveness and efficiency of health systems to cope with the increase of elderly NCD patients. This 'demographic time bomb' can readily justify austerity or cost-saving measures such as the ones put forward by the European Semester: in the closer alignment between the ESIF and the European Semester, the priority for health-related investments is put on financial sustainability of health systems, requiring modernisation, tech innovation and community-based health-care with a view to fostering healthy, active and autonomous ageing. Member states who want to benefit from ESIF money for health need to demonstrate how the investment fits into a broader modernisation of health system strategy which improves cost-effectiveness:

> In the 2014-2020 programming period, health infrastructure investments and other investments in health in individual Member States are supported mostly as an integral part of their health system reforms in order to ensure that the system is effective and efficient. For this purpose, Member States using ESIF as a source of funding for their health systems had to present a strategic framework for health investments; every investment had to be in line with this framework. (European Commission, 2016a, p. 16)

[9] 'Future-proofing' is a term also used in the Better Regulation documents (European Commission, 2017b, p. 149).

While it is difficult to argue against 'health system effectiveness and efficiency' as a desirable goal, it is important to bear in mind the underlying normative assumptions that drive the meaning of what represents 'effectiveness and efficiency'. The European Semester CSR for health are not designed by public health experts but are designed with a view to reducing national spending on health. 'Effectiveness and efficiency', in this context, refers more to cost-saving and responsibilisation of individuals.

Portraying the growing wave of elderly people as a threat to the financial sustainability of health systems downplays and even obscures the evidence that exists on the link between NCDs and inequities and precludes the possibility to consider structural changes to improve public health. The CSR published in 2019 in the frame of the European Semester largely revolves around three main themes: ensuring financial sustainability of the pension and healthcare system, which in many cases also explicitly means raising the age of retirement and cracking down on early retirement (see, e.g., CSR for Austria, Portugal, Czech Republic, Poland, Romania, Slovakia, Ireland, Italy, Slovenia, Luxembourg, Finland and Belgium).[10] A second theme is to reduce unemployment by cracking down on incentives to remain out of work (see, e.g., Finland and Germany) as well as by creating incentives specially for women, vulnerable people, low-skilled people and migrants (Portugal, Belgium, Netherlands, Czech Republic, Hungary, Ireland, Slovenia and Austria). Finally, another of the common themes of the 2019 CSRs is to create a more business-friendly environment, with recommended mechanisms like improving stakeholder consultation, reducing regulatory burden and competition, and favouring economic investment in areas like research and innovation (see, e.g., CSRs for Portugal, Poland, Belgium, Czech Republic, Italy, Slovenia, Austria, Luxembourg and Bulgaria). However, the public spending cuts put forward to ensure the financial sustainability of health systems 'in an ageing population' (i.e. reducing unemployment and pension spending) is likely to increase inequities that worsen population health. Neoliberal austerity measures, such as notably ones following the Eurozone crisis, have been associated with a deterioration of population

[10] 2019 Country Specific Recommendations can be found here: https://ec.europa.eu/info/publications/2019-european-semester-country-specific-recommendations-commission-recommendations_en.

health (Karanikolos et al., 2013; Kentikelenis et al., 2011; McKee et al., 2017; Stuckler et al., 2017).

Economic and Biomedical Paradigms: Personalised Medicine as the Solution

A second implication of the 'ageing population' framing of NCDs is the solution mostly located in market innovation. Here we have an interaction between the economic and the biomedical paradigm of health. This framing does not spark reflection on the macrosocial determinants of health, precisely because it presents the rise of NCDs as the result of 'how well' the current system functions given the life expectancy improvements. Placing the cause of NCDs on ageing then favours technological solutions at the level of the individual rather than favouring social solutions at the level of society. This, in turn, also mobilises the 'health as a market' face of the economic paradigm, insofar as solutions are thought to lie in industry innovations—medical devices, new pharmaceuticals, but also mobile apps for self-management, to name a few. If the NCD 'crisis' is perceived as the result of ageing population and not of a more deep-seated problem of neoliberal capitalism, then this crisis can be resolved using the usual, market-creating approach. In other words, in a framing driven by a combination of biomedical and economic paradigms of health, the solutions naturally ought to be sought in the realm of biomedical and technological innovation. This type of solution also strengthens the justification for more health innovation as a means to 'empower' people to manage themselves (e.g. with smartphone apps) and remain autonomous—ultimately to ensure they remain out of the hospital.

> The narrative is shifting more towards personalised medicine, using tech for kinds of personalised nutrition, personalised medicine etc. [...] Nothing against personalised medicine but there should be a population approach too, it should be within a framework for the population. (Quoted from interviewee 13)

This quote from a health advocate critiques precisely the trend, in relation to NCDs, to turn towards personalised medicine and personalised nutrition, i.e. effectively the creation of a new market, rather than to think about approaches to public health that put the population—not the individual—at the centre (Rose, 1985; McLaren et al., 2010). The absence of population-wide rationale is visible, for example, in the fact that the SGPP has created a subgroup at the request of the EIB to investigate the cost-effectiveness of a particular high-tech cancer treatment, despite the fact that the SGPP is supposed to be about health promotion, disease prevention and NCD management.

The rationale linking ageing population, NCDs, personalised medicine and the economic paradigm of health is well encapsulated in Juncker's Commissioner for Research, Science and Innovation Carlos Moedas's publication compellingly entitled 'Better Health for All – one person at a time' (2016[11]). The publication argues that '[w]ith an ageing population and a growing number of chronic diseases, Europe needs to change its healthcare paradigm. Personalised medicine holds the promise of bringing about change' (second paragraph). It then goes on to explain how personalised medicine can lead to better health of individuals, as well as economic growth resulting from all the potential for innovation that lies in this field. A large part of EU research funding on the topic of health is spent on developing personalised medicine, with an allocated €872 million for the 2014–2017 period[12] (European Commission, 2017h). The point is to combine health improvement in the context of NCDs and chronic diseases, with economic growth and innovation. The notion that these advancements are unlikely to address, or may even worsen, underlying health determinants—most importantly socioeconomic inequities—is not a perspective that is engaged with.

Lastly, another EC priority in the field of NCDs is to develop and innovate in health apps (these can include healthy lifestyle promoting apps or chronic condition management apps, for example), telemedicine and health information portals. On the one hand, this is seen as a way to ensure patient/people's autonomy and minimise their burden on health systems. At the same time, it is also seen as a way to keep these people in the workforce and keep them contributing to the economy. And finally, these tools also represent a data mine worth exploiting:

> Patient and user-generated health and care data are expected to further proliferate in the coming decade, creating continuously evolving and learning health systems. This could potentially disrupt the established

[11] Accessed 12 November 2019. Available from: https://ec.europa.eu/commission/commissioners/2014-2019/moedas/blog/better-health-all-one-person-time_en.

[12] Out of €7.4 billion (see European Commission, 2013c).

> status quo of health and social care delivery, opening up the ability to deliver more targeted health and social care services to citizens, and unlocking opportunities for new, data-driven economic models in public and consumer markets. (European Commission, 2018c, p. 45)

The point here is not to negate the desirability of keeping people autonomous as long as possible. Rather, the problem lies with the framing that emphasises the NCDs crisis as the inevitable result of an increase in life expectancy, which warrants technological innovation, self-management tools and budget cuts. Indeed, life expectancy increases are not uniform and mask growing inequities (Burström et al., 2005; Singh & Siapush, 2006) which are left unacknowledged by this framing (and, even when acknowledged along with ageing, the interpretation of health inequality still fails to lead to thinking about societal transformation, as will be outlined below). Another point that this framing brings to the forefront is the interaction between the biomedical paradigm of health and the economic one. The biomedical paradigm of health pushes in the direction of individualised solutions, while the economic one pushes towards market innovation. Both together lead to a situation where personalised medicine is most invested in, at the expense of population-wide approaches.

Personalised solutions to NCDs also aligns with the behavioural paradigm of health, given that it aims to give people (especially elder people) the tools to manage themselves independently. Admittedly, this is a desirable goal as such, only it is couched in a discourse that prioritises economic growth over population wellbeing. Therefore, it is debatable whether the actual concern the policy aims to address is people's wellbeing or instead limit potential increases of public spending. This distinction is important because the latter is likely to be blind to differences in accessibility (in a broad sense) of innovations, and in turn risks exacerbating inequities in health. Most importantly, aiming to keep people autonomous for the sake of saving money rather than out of concern for health and wellbeing is counterproductive, because it is often accompanied with cost-saving, austerity measures that negatively affect macrosocial determinants of health.

The 'ageing population' framing of NCDs, in turn, can be seen as shaped by the economic paradigm of health, together with the security and the biomedical paradigm. This discursive constellation does not allow to move away from the ultimate priority, which is to foster economic growth, by producing health innovations. At the same time, it also legitimises cost-saving measures. However, disciplining people to remain autonomous by using these innovative gadgets is not a sustainable strategy to meaningfully prioritise public health, when taken alongside cost-saving measures that tend to worsen socioeconomic determinants of health. This whole web of interaction between health paradigms and NCD frames represents part of the neoliberal background ideational structures prevailing in the EU context which undermine the possibilities for HiAP uptake.

6.3 The Positivist Paradigm of Knowledge

The previous section has looked at paradigms and frames of health to better understand what kinds of background ideational obstacles, related to how *health* is made sense of, stand in the way of a meaningful HiAP uptake at EU level. The dominant paradigms, and the frames that stem from them, tend to be underpinned by neoliberal rationality, and undermine the possibility to think of a normative, social equity focused HiAP. To further investigate the background ideational structures that prevail in the EU, their relationship to neoliberalism and how they constrain or undermine HiAP, it is also worth looking at paradigms and frames of *knowledge*. The insights gained from the in-depth semi-structured elite interviews steered the attention towards the epistemology of HiAP, and the dilemma between appealing to normative neutrality and explicit values-based advocacy. The way that knowledge is made sense of, the legitimation of certain types of knowledge over others, and the definition of what constitutes 'evidence' is normative, relates to 'power *in* ideas', and has important implications for HiAP, as will be shown in the remainder of this chapter.

What is more, the role of knowledge and evidence in the EC, and especially in DG SANTE, is of particular salience: given its propensity to act within the realm of 'soft governance', knowledge gathering, collecting and monitoring of data, commitments to evidence-based practice in public health, good and best practices, are all strong themes in DG SANTE.[13] Knowledge and evidence are a red thread that runs through DG SANTE's activities and expresses itself in different ways: in relation

[13] Source: interviewees 3, 7, 23 and 28.

to the objective of protecting EU citizens from health threats, knowledge is referred to in the sense of monitoring, data gathering by member states to be compiled and processed at EC level (Flear, 2015). The health system modernisation goal also relies much on knowledge, as it taps into the scope for collaborative innovation in health tech, but also in health research, especially on rare diseases, where EU added value is perceived to be highest. When it comes to health determinants, the knowledge emphasis manifests in the facilitation of sharing best practices between member states. A common position, with respect to NCD prevention and health promotion, is that much knowledge and evidence regarding NCDs already exists, and that now it is a matter of processing it and making it accessible to policymakers (European Commission, n.d.a). The role of DG SANTE in health promotion and NCD prevention, in turn, has become very much targeted at supporting member states by providing them a choice of scientifically and rigorously selected best practices.

Some initiatives of DG SANTE that encapsulate its role as a knowledge broker very well include, for example, the 'State of health in the EU' cycle (European Commission, n.d.b). The 'State of health in the EU' is a two-year cycle throughout which the EC, together with the European Observatory on Health Systems and Policies, and the member states, provides health intelligence for member states, in order to support their evidence-based best practices implementation in the area of health (European Commission, 2017a, 2017f, 2018d). Another example would be the ECHI (formerly called European Community Health indicators, see: European Commission, 2013b). ECHI is an initiative aimed at better integrating health data management across member states. The size of the section of the EU research budget dedicated to 'health, demographic change and wellbeing' also reflects the importance of the health intelligence and knowledge production role of the EC.[14] The EC research agenda is not limited to funding research and complementing the budgets of member states, but it also plays a coordination role (Greer et al., 2014). The HP funds multiple types of research projects in the area of health

[14] The research budget for the 2014–2020 programming period is called 'Horizon 2020' and amounts to EUR 80 billion. Out of this sum, 38.53% is dedicated to the broad section called 'societal challenges', and within that section, almost EUR 7.5 billion is dedicated to the sub-section 'health, demographic change and wellbeing' (European Commission, 2013c). The largest part of the remaining subsection under 'societal challenges' is relevant to environmental research and sustainable future, which also relates to health.

promotion and NCD prevention, including joint actions such as 'JANPA' (Joint Action on Nutrition and Physical Activity[15]) and 'CHRODIS+'[16] on the topic of chronic diseases and which is now geared towards implementing good practices. The CHRODIS+ website links to DG SANTE's best practice portal for public health. Finally, the SGPP can also be considered an initiative representative of DG SANTE's knowledge broker role. One interviewee summarises the role of the EC in health promotion and NCD prevention in this way:

> They [the EC] are moving from member states should should should [sic] do this, to much more something like 'here's what's working in one country' and promoting the good practice as it is. [...] it was really about identifying what is their [the EC] role in the determinants of health side of SANTE, what is their [the EC] role and how can they foster member state's national regional local level taking up initiatives that actually work and have an impact. [...] The idea was to sit down and have some criteria say how can we measure how good a practice is. And what are the priorities? So, the focus was very much on evidence of outputs, outcomes, impact. [...] It wasn't for us to say for example 'in food reformulation, industry self-regulation obviously doesn't work, so we need to legislate or whatever'. That wasn't so much the point of our discussions. (Quoted from interviewee 23)

Evidence-Based Policymaking

As suggested above, DG SANTE puts a strong emphasis on adopting and proposing 'evidence-based' policies. The concept of evidence-based policymaking was preceded by and aims to emulate, the principles of evidence-based medicine (EBM) (Parkhurst & Abeysinghe, 2016). EBM is embedded in the positivist research paradigm characteristic of applied natural sciences. It traditionally regards randomised controlled trials as the gold standard and most reliable type of evidence (Nutley et al., 2013). The adequacy of transposing this approach to social policy, however, is highly contentious and is being criticised in a growing body of literature (Bacchi, 2009, 2012; Bache, 2019; Greenhalgh & Russell, 2009; Marston & Watts, 2003; Neylan, 2008; Parkhurst, 2017; Petticrew &

[15] See: http://www.janpa.eu/.

[16] See: http://chrodis.eu/.

Roberts, 2003; Sanderson, 2006; Smith, 2013). It has been argued that this understanding of evidence is not useful when dealing with complex, 'wicked' problems such as climate change (Dryzek, 1990; Parkhurst, 2017; Sanderson, 2006), and indeed public health (Kickbusch, 1989), and wellbeing (Bache et al., 2016).

The notion of evidence-based policymaking, then, is far from unproblematic. The accent put on using scientific language in politics—technocratic discourse—has been criticised for 'us[ing] the apparent objectivity of scientific discourse for [...] presenting "highly contentious" statements as "uncontentious"' (McKenna & Graham, 2000, p. 224; see also Fairclough, 2003). In the UK, it has been associated in the UK with Blair's third way, 'post-ideological' approach to public policy (Bache, 2019; Ferlie & McGivern, 2014). This approach to policymaking needs to be contextualised in the 'new public management' reforms that occurred in the 1990s and which saw the public sector becoming increasingly closely modelled on business management, both in terms of its organisation and activity and in terms of language used (Lane, 2000). The new public management wave has been followed by a turn to 'network governance', which facilitates the creation of multi-sectoral, multistakeholder partnerships and collaborations to reconnect the previously devolved, privatised or contracted out competencies (Bevir, 2011; Ferlie & McGivern, 2014). New public management can be seen as part of the neoliberal agenda as it represents a typical example of intrusion of market rationality in non-market spheres (Bevir, 2011; Christensen & Laegreid, 2007). They echo the points raised about EU NMG and governmentality.

Parkhurst (2017) categorises two main types of problem that follow from the transposition of an EBM approach to public policymaking. The first one relates to the risk of depoliticising politics; the reduction of inherently political and value laden policies, to objective, apolitical issues that can be addressed in a technical way. This obscures underlying norms and values that are inevitably present in policies and shuts down possibilities for dialogue around these norms. This is what he refers to as 'issue bias'. The second type of bias described by Parkhurst relates to the risk of politicisation of science, the instrumental (mis)use of scientific evidence for political ends—'technical bias' (Parkhurst, 2017). An instance of technical bias was described earlier in relation to the tobacco industry, the Better Regulation agenda and the precautionary principle.

This section here is more concerned with the depoliticising effects of the positivist knowledge paradigm, as representing power *in* ideas.

Indeed, this knowledge paradigm implies a very narrow and limited, instrumental view of the research/policy relationship. However, possible research utilisation is far from limited to an instrumentalist view of research 'filling a knowledge gap' and providing ready-to-use solutions to problems (Weiss, 1979). The research/policy relationship can also be a more fluid one of awareness raising, where theoretical perspectives slowly inform different ways to make sense of issues, potentially redefining policy agenda in the long run (Weiss, 1977).

Evidence as conceptualised within a positivist, hypothetico-deductive paradigm of knowledge excludes these other possible relationships between research and policy, and consequently excludes several other kinds of evidence. Not all research evidence fits into the positivist knowledge paradigm. Some of the literature investigating the links between neoliberalism and ill-health reviewed in Chapter Two, for example, does not feature in DG SANTE's evidence collection and processing. This echoes Smith and Joyce's (2012) finding that while policymakers in the UK working on health inequality were familiar with the arguments put forward by Marmot or Wilkinson and Pickett, this evidence was unlikely to be featured in policy (Smith, 2014; Smith & Joyce, 2012). Furthermore, there exists evidence demonstrating the lack of effectiveness of industry self-regulation in relation to obesity in a manner that fits into the positivist paradigm (see Ronit & Jensen, 2014), yet arguably it would be difficult for DG SANTE to use this kind of evidence, because it does not fit with the EC's official line according to which the first choice should always be to encourage self-regulation. More normatively explicit 'politics of health' research that lies outside of the dominant knowledge paradigm—such as the literature building on Marxist and Gramscian theories, or feminist or post-modern theories—are entirely absent from the debate in DG SANTE. What becomes clear is that DG SANTE's inclination to evidence-based policymaking presupposes a particular type of ready-to-use evidence, which is deemed as obvious and objective, but it excludes research evidence that does not meet these particular paradigmatic requirements.

6.4 'SMART' Framing of Evidence

Now it is worth delving deeper and analysing the dominant framing of evidence, by looking at the various EU HPs and their evolution. EU HPs outline the strategic direction of the involvement of the EU in public health for a given financial period. So far, there have been three HPs (1st HP from 2003 to 2008; 2nd HP from 2008 to 2013; 3rd HP from 2014 to 2020). The evolution of the HPs is quite clear: they went from putting forward a small number of broad objectives and strong normative commitments to public health, to a large number of increasingly specific, measurable objectives and with less and less reference to normative commitments (European Commission, 2007; European Union, 2002, 2014). This evidence frame will be referred to hereinafter as 'SMART evidence'. The SMART acronym, which refers to specific, measurable, achievable, relevant and time-bound, was created in the early 1980s and most prominently used in business and management to rationally guide decision-making and project evaluations among other things (Britt Bjerke & Renger, 2017; Goodwin & Wright, 2004, pp. 27–70). As such, the uptake of the SMART approach in public policy can be seen as a consequence of the rise of new public management in the 90s, where business approaches have been imported into the public policy sphere. The evolution towards SMART evidence is best described in the Q&A document accompanying the establishment of the 3rd HP:

Box 6.1 'How does the third health programme compare with the previous two?' (European Commission, 2014d)

"The new programme is more focused towards how health can contribute to growth and to the objectives of Europe 2020 - in particular as regards employment, innovation, sustainability. It is also more focused on key issues where EU action can deliver added value and make a real difference to Member States.

Priorities are better defined and more targeted, with a focus on 23 key thematic priorities that address current health challenges.

There are clear indicators to monitor the progress made against the objectives and to regularly review the programme priorities. Improvements in knowledge and information sharing mechanisms will lead to better decision making in health policies at regional, national and European level. Better dissemination of results will help Member States and the health community to make better use of action under the programme. [...]"

This evolution towards defining narrow, measurable objectives and away from broader commitments is a result of the mid-term and ex-post evaluations of the first two HPs. Both the first and second HP evaluations identified the lack of SMART objectives as a major weakness (European

Commission, 2008, 2011a, 2011b, 2015a; European Court of Auditors, 2009).

The second HP had the strongest emphasis on HiAP (it was established not long after the Finnish HiAP presidency), but the mid-term and ex-post evaluations provided a sober account of the extent to which HiAP, as an element of DG SANTE's integrated health strategy, had been taken up in the EC (European Commission, 2011c). The executive summary of the mid-term evaluation of the second HP suggested that the health strategy was not successful in mainstreaming the health norms and values in other EC policy areas (p. 6). Thereafter, mentions of health-related values and norms were largely dropped, and priorities became streamlined more explicitly with the Europe 2020 strategy for growth, competitiveness and investment (European Commission, 2015a).

The third HP is considered a major improvement and better value for money (European Commission, 2017g). The objectives on health promotion and NCD prevention (operational objective number 1) are still considered too broad and not clearly defined enough, and the mid-term evaluation recommends that, while this topic should not be dropped altogether, its EU added value should be made clearer and more defined, given the breadth of the topic (European Commission, 2017g, p. 35). The report stresses that, in the area of health promotion, the single most important EU added value is the sharing of knowledge—very clearly recommending that this is where the EC needs to concentrate its efforts in the area of health promotion.

Over the last years, DG SANTE has put much effort into streamlining the programme's objectives and improving its coherence.[17] As the public health approach in the EC was becoming more streamlined and coherent, the language of the health programmes became increasingly oriented towards setting out SMART objectives. The most striking evolution in HPs is the shift from few, broad and strongly normative objectives in the first and second health programme, towards many, narrow and SMART objectives in the third health programme. Along with this process, normative references were dropped, as broad HiAP objectives were not perceived to produce these types of measurable results. Instead, DG SANTE became more focused on its knowledge brokering role, which is perceived as the only EU added value in the field of

[17] Source: interviewees 3, 7 and 8.

health promotion and NCD prevention. Relatedly, demonstrating EU added value follows similar criteria of 'objective measurability'. Along with focusing on SMART evidence, the notion of 'EU added value' as a crucial determinant of EU level action has become increasingly important (European Commission, 2017g, 2018e). CHAFEA has elaborated a formalised 'EU added value score' from 1 to 10 to evaluate potential funding under the third Health Programme (European Commission, 2017g). This suggests that EU added value should be objectively quantifiable, along the lines of a technical rationale. CHAFEA streamlines seven EU added value criteria: best practice and knowledge exchange; benchmarking; (multistakeholder) network building; addressing cross-border threats; health issues where the internal market is strongly concerned (e.g. patient mobility); innovation in healthcare; and optimising the use financial resources (avoiding duplications).

SMART evidence reflects a conceptualisation of evidence as objectively measurable, aligned with a positivist, hypothetico-deductive knowledge paradigm. This framing of evidence also has a strong appeal to being apolitical, objective, quantitatively measurable and discrete in isolating a causal relationship (A can be isolated as the factor/one of the factors, that caused B). Going back to the State of health in the EU cycle, the emphasis is put on the neutrality of the information given. Indeed, the cycle's purpose is stated as 'to inform and support policymaking, not to make recommendations' (European Commission, n.d.b). It is stated that 'the report which is published every two years provides a neutral, descriptive comparison of all EU countries on the basis of publicly available data and indicators' (European Commission, n.d.c).

Why is this important, and what are the implications of SMART evidence frame for HiAP? The sections below will make the case that this frame, rooted in the positivist knowledge paradigm which is itself underpinned by neoliberal rationality, precludes a focus on the social and normative dimensions of health necessary to adopt HiAP (Bambra et al., 2005; Smith, 2013; Ståhl et al., 2006). Two problematic elements are developed in this section: on the one hand, SMART evidence's (inevitably failing) attempt to break down complexity into discrete, measurable components, and on the other hand, the problematic appeal to normative neutrality of SMART evidence.

Attempts to Break Down Complexity

While HiAP is about recognising the complexity of determinants of health, the dominant meaning of legitimate evidence as SMART thwarts any embrace of complexity by attempting to categorise health determinants into discrete variables causally related to health outcomes. Indeed, the central idea of the SMART approach in management decision-making has been described as 'by splitting the problem into small parts and focusing on each part separately, the decision maker was likely to acquire a better understanding of his or her problem than would have been achieved by taking a holistic view' (Goodwin & Wright, 2004, p. 57).

Complexity of public health determinants is seen as a considerable challenge within DG SANTE. One way to illustrate these irreconcilable characteristics around complexity is to go back to the ECHI and look at them more closely. As one interviewee explained, it is very difficult to set out a list of discrete health indicators:

> [...] when you think of the EU you think of standardised, very strict standardised data collection that applies for a limited number of indicators. A good example is if you look at employment you have four or five key indicators that are used at EU level [...] In health we were never able to reach that degree of lightness, so we started with something like a couple of thousands of indicators, and now we have a short list that is under 100. But even under 100 is not four [...] (Quoted from interviewee 7)

The ECHI list aims to single out HiAP as a separate 'policy area' category, which is further broken down into 'Health in All Policies (HIAP) including occupational and environmental health' (see: Appendix 1—European Commission, n.d.d). Given the awareness of the importance of HiAP, the ECHI aim to include that 'variable' as a separate policy area, to which the various other indicators may have relevance. The only indicators identified as HiAP relevant, however, are those pertaining to occupational health and to environmental health. While including HiAP in the ECHI grid is likely to stem from a concern and awareness of the importance of HiAP, narrowing it to a separate, discrete variable negates the complexity that a HiAP approach is about. An indicator like 'vegetable consumption', despite its clear relevance to both agricultural and trade policies, is not marked as HiAP relevant in this set up. This does not mean that policymakers from DG SANTE do not recognise the relevance of agricultural policies for health, but these types of classifications contribute to shaping the meaning of HiAP. In this case, a narrow, artificial classification confines 'HiAP' into meaning occupational and environmental health. While occupational and environmental health are all relevant areas for HiAP, all other policy areas are relevant too. Another example relates to the Best Practice Portal search engine. When selecting 'Health in All Policies' and 'Health in All Policies Actions', 12 initiatives are listed (as of 3 July 2019). Five out of the 12 projects listed as HiAP Best Practices are projects which have as their main objective changing individuals' behaviours towards healthy nutrition and physical activity by educating and raising awareness.[18] The attempt, driven by SMART evidence, to classify what represents HiAP best practice, seems to lead back to more proximal determinants of health (such as individual behaviour). This, again, reduces HiAP and shapes its meaning in ways which obscure the complexity HiAP is supposed to take into account.

As explained by an interviewee who contributed to the 2006 Finnish Presidency priorities, HiAP cannot be thought of as a separate entity at all, because it represents 'a way of working'. Trying to isolate a discrete 'HiAP' category is problematic, because it narrows the HiAP scope and fails to adequately take into account the complexity that the HiAP concept illustrates an understanding of.[19] Attempting to isolate HiAP as a separate variable or category, which reflects a SMART evidence logic, stifles and narrows down the meaning of HiAP to associate it to what seems most easily measurable. One interviewee argued that 'there is an understanding of complexity, but complexity is used against action' (Quoted from interviewee 13). This idea is interesting because it goes right to the heart of the epistemological tension in public health research, and what counts as legitimate evidence: complexity of causal links can be strategically invoked to argue that a policy/law/regulation would never be able to solve the problem. Indeed, the notion of complexity has been instrumentalised by the food industry to bring the focus back onto individual behaviour, arguing that public health policies are too simplistic given the uniquely complex context of each individual (Petticrew et al., 2017; Savona et al., 2020). In a space where action needs to be informed by narrow, SMART evidence, it becomes easy to dismiss the

[18] The best practice portal can be found under: https://webgate.ec.europa.eu/dyna/bp-portal/index_search.cfm.

[19] Source: interviewee 32.

areas of action that are perceived as too complex, regardless of how important and necessary the issues at hand. What this interviewee critiques are the multiple mid-term evaluations of the various health programmes, which consistently pushed the programme away from tackling the most important public health issues, i.e. NCDs.

Appeal to Normative Neutrality

With its root in the positivist hypothetico-deductive knowledge paradigm, the SMART evidence frame strongly appeals to normative neutrality, and this undermines the potential for an explicitly normative HiAP vision. HiAP is in essence a normative concept, underpinned by values of social justice, solidarity, human rights and a will to prioritise population health and wellbeing over economic growth. The explicit normativity of HiAP does not preclude a strong rootedness in scientific rigour. However, such a stance tends to be put 'in opposition' to a more neutral, objective and non-ideological status quo. Normative neutrality, especially in social issues like health, is not achievable, and any claim to normative neutrality hides underpinning values that are merely taken for granted or seen as unavoidable.

One telling example of apparent normative neutrality and its synergy with SMART evidence is the case of health inequalities (see Smith, 2013). The concept of health inequalities is very much present in the mainstream EC and DG SANTE debate. However, the points made by critical social scientists that socioeconomic inequities are detrimental to health and wellbeing not only of the poorer population groups, but even for the wealthy, too, and therefore require a societal solution rather than an individually targeted one (Wilkinson & Pickett, 2010), are absent from DG SANTE evidence talks. Constructing SMART evidence on the topic of health inequities leads to the tendency to think of inequities as a measurable gap, with the aim to bring people from the bottom to the top, with measurable results (Smith, 2013). The issue is that this conflates poverty and inequity, and results in targeting poor people and acting upon narrowly defined 'risk factors' rather than changing societal structures (Glasgow & Schrecker, 2016; Smith, 2013). Going even further, the language of 'health inequality' itself can be seen as problematic, because it medicalises and thereby contributes to depoliticising what are essentially socioeconomic inequalities (Lynch, 2020). HiAP thinking about health inequities would identify the roots of health inequities in socioeconomic inequities and would lead to fundamental changes towards building a more equal society, which would include, at the very least, a vast redistribution of wealth. This explicit normativity clashes with the framing of SMART evidence, according to which the rationale of singling out vulnerable groups with specific measures aimed at quantifiably reducing the gap between them and the wealthier population, is (mistakenly) accepted as being normatively neutral, objective.

Many health actors are uncomfortable steering the discussion towards the political roots of inequalities, precisely because it is perceived as too ideological, when the expectation is that health needs to remain 'beyond ideologies':

> [...] schemes targeted at poor people are not going to solve the inequality issue. They can cut some of the sharpest edges, but it still leaves you with the whole macroeconomic policy. And this is something that health actors are not comfortable talking about. [...] Targeted measures should be seen as a phase-out. [...] This whole discussion is something that health actors are not comfortable going into, because it's seen as too far removed. [...] On the other hand, industry likes to say 'it's not an issue of tobacco/alcohol/soda etc... it's an issue of poverty' in order to shift responsibility. And proving that they, as multinational corporations, are responsible for the poverty, is very difficult: try to make that argument, you'll be labelled an ideologue, it's difficult to make a water-tight case. (Quoted from interviewee 13)

The argument here is that SMART evidence is normative—rather than neutral—and that, with its embeddedness in a positivist knowledge paradigm, it is easily aligned with neoliberalism. The normatively neutral veneer of the SMART evidence frame means that the HiAP normativity appears as unreasonably ideological in comparison. SMART evidence also tends to lead to the type of data gathering and evidence which relates to cost/cost-saving estimates, given that these are obvious measurables. In turn, policy rationales are also geared towards what leads to easily measurable results, i.e. financially quantifiable results (Parkhurst, 2017). As put by Koivusalo (2010, p. 501): 'In reporting on HiAP we tend to seek assessment on what works rather than what should be done and how to get there'.

6.5 Conclusion: HiAP and the EU Background Ideational Web

This chapter has turned towards the prevailing 'background ideational structures' in the EU, focusing on the power *in* ideas. In order to dig into these background cognitive and normative elements, it used the 'framework for analysing global health policy-making' proposed by Rushton and Williams (2012), linking neoliberal core, paradigms and frames.

The first half of the chapter has looked at paradigms and frames related to health and NCDs. It introduced the economic paradigm of health, i.e. seeing health as an investment with good returns, as well as a profitable market in which innovation can lead to economic growth. The 'ageing population' framing of NCDs presents characteristics that stem from the interactions between the economic paradigm of health, together with the security and the biomedical paradigms of health. Indeed, this framing of NCDs leads to constructing the growing ageing population as a security threat, posed by a wave of chronically ill, elderly people, to the financial sustainability of health systems. This justifies cost-saving measures; the goal being to decrease public spending by disciplining ageing people into managing their conditions autonomously (and, if possible, to also remain active contributors in the labour market). Solutions to this 'crisis' are not identified in the potential for changing the political system; instead, they are located in the realm of more market creation, in line with neoliberal capitalism. These new market solutions, which include the rise of personalised medicine, and the turn towards digital solutions (e-Health, m-Health), are driven by both the economic and biomedical paradigm of health.

By focusing on rising life expectancy, ultimately this framing implies that the NCDs 'crisis' is (at least in part), the result of progress. This assumption tacitly endorses the prevailing system (which after all has led to said progress) and in turn prevents any fundamental questioning of the political and ideological system that in large part is responsible for the rise of NCDs—i.e. neoliberal capitalism. Rather, it embraces its methods, such as austerity and market innovation.

The second half of this chapter explored the dominant paradigms and frames of knowledge in the EU and their implications for HiAP. After justifying the necessity to look at knowledge paradigms and frames of evidence, it explained how the evidence-based policymaking approach that dominates in DG SANTE is rooted in a positivist, hypothetico-deductive knowledge paradigm typically associated with applied STEM subjects (science, technology, engineering and maths) and medicine ('evidence-based medicine'). However, issues emerge when transposing the EBM logic to policymaking. Delving further into the specific framing of evidence and how it developed along the different HPs, this chapter examined the use of SMART evidence, where legitimate evidence is specific, measurable, achievable, relevant and time-bound. The SMART evidence frame, however, has problematic implications for HiAP. Firstly, SMART evidence pushes towards a Cartesian breakdown of complex problems into sub-problems to be tackled 'separately' as a means to solve the whole problem. This is fundamentally at odds with the HiAP logic which advocates for an embrace of complexity. Secondly, SMART evidence appeals to normative neutrality and objectivity, whereas HiAP requires an explicit engagement with norms and values.

Here we need to draw attention to the importance of the politics of knowledge. Neoliberal rationality can permeate even in how knowledge is made sense of. The positivist knowledge paradigm, while it need not intrinsically be 'neoliberal', can often be aligned with this ideology and perpetuate it in subtle ways. This is visible in the relationship between the positivist knowledge paradigm and the SMART evidence framing, and how it affects the possibility to promote HiAP.

Paradigms and frames can be seen as parts of a cross-cutting ideational system that reinforce each other and weave the cognitive background that structures individuals' sense-making. They are not neutral, pre-existing, but as this chapter has shown, they contain normative assumptions, which, in the cases looked at herein, reproduce neoliberal rationality and undermine HiAP. The question remains: Is it possible to exploit dominant paradigms and change them 'from within', make them work *for* HiAP advocates? Indeed, while certain background ideational structures dominate in a particular institutional context, it does not mean that they go unrecognised by individuals working within these institutions, who may even be critical (or not) of these paradigms and frames. Relatedly, ideational structures are not immutable and have become ingrained, taken-for-granted over time also through active social construction and agency. In short, background ideational structures can be challenged and can evolve, even though this evolution is likely to be very slow. These potential spaces for contestation are explored in the next chapter. They may lie perhaps not so much in changing the EU institutional architecture, but in contesting dominant power *in* ideas, gradually changing their meanings, using power *over* and *through* ideas.

References

Ayo, N. (2012). Understanding health promotion in a neoliberal climate and the making of health conscious citizens. *Critical Public Health., 22*(1), 99–105.

Bacchi, C. (2009). *Analyzing policy: What's the problem represented to be?* Pearson.

Bacchi, C. (2012). Why study problematizations? Making the politics visible. *Open Journal of Political Science, 2*(1), 1–8.

Bache, I. (2019). How does evidence matter? Understanding 'what works' for wellbeing. *Social Indicators Research, 142*, 1153–1173.

Bache, I., Reardon, L., & Anand, P. (2016). Wellbeing as a wicked problem: Navigating the arguments for the role of government. *Journal of Happiness Studies, 17*, 893–912.

Bambra, C., Fox, D., & Scott-Samuel, A. (2005). Towards a politics of health. *Health Promotion International, 20*(2), 187–193.

Baum, F., & Fisher, M. (2014). Why behavioural health promotion endures despite its failure to reduce health inequities. *Sociology of Health and Illness, 36*(2), 213–225.

Benson, C., & Glasgow, S. (2015). Noncommunicable diseases as a security issue. In S. Rushton & J. Youde (Eds.), *Routledge handbook of global health security* (pp. 175–186). Routledge.

Bevir, M. (2011). Governance and governmentality after neoliberalism. *Policy & Politics, 39*(4), 457–471.

Burström, K., Johannesson, M., & Didrichsen, F. (2005). Increasing socio-economic inequalities in life expectancy and QALYs in Sweden 1980–1997. *Health Economics, 14*(8), 831–850.

Britt Bjerke, M., & Renger, R. (2017). Being smart about writing SMART objectives. *Evaluation and Program Planning, 61*, 125–127.

Christensen, T., & Laegreid, P. (2007). (Eds.). Introduction—Theoretical approach and research questions. In *Transcending new public management: The transformation of public sector reforms*. Ashgate.

Dryzek, J. S. (1990). *Discursive democracy: Politics, policy and political science*. Cambridge University Press.

Elbe, S. (2006). Should HIV/AIDS be securitized? The ethical dilemmas of linking HIV/ AIDS and security. *International Studies Quarterly, 50*(1), 119–144.

European Commission. (2000). Communication from the Commission to the Council, the European Parliament, the Economic and Social Committee and the Committee of the Regions on the health strategy of the European Community (COM/2000/0285 final). https://eur-lex.europa.eu/legal-content/EN/TXT/?uri=CELEX%3A52000DC0285. Accessed 12 November 2019.

European Commission. (2007). *Together for health: A strategic approach for the EU 2008–2013* [White Paper]. Brussels, 23 October. COM(2007) 630 final. https://eur-lex.europa.eu/legal-content/EN/TXT/PDF/?uri=CELEX:52007DC0630&from=EN. Accessed 12 November 2019.

European Commission. (2008, July 24). Interim evaluation of the implementation of the Public Health Programme (2003–2008) [Communication from the Commission to the European Parliament, The Council, The European Economic and Social Committee and the Committee of the Regions] Brussels. COM(2008) 484 final. https://eur-lex.europa.eu/legal-content/EN/TXT/PDF/?uri=CELEX:52008DC0484&from=EN. Accessed 12 November 2019.

European Commission. (2009, October 20). *Solidarity in health: Reducing health inequalities in the EU* [Communication from the Commission to the European Parliament, the Council, the European Economic and Social Committee and the Committee of the Regions] Brussels. COM(2009) 567 final. https://ec.europa.eu/health/ph_determinants/socio_economics/documents/com2009_en.pdf. Accessed 12 November 2019.

European Commission. (2011a). *Mid-term evaluation of the health strategy 2008–2013 Final Report*. Report prepared by "Public Health Evaluation and Impact Assessment Consortium" (PHEIAC). https://ec.europa.eu/health/sites/health/files/programme/docs/mthp_final_report_oct2011_en.pdf. Accessed 12 November 2019.

European Commission. (2011b, March). *Ex-post evaluation of the Public Health Programme (PHP) 2003–2008 Final report* [Prepared by COWI]. https://ec.europa.eu/health/sites/health/files/programme/docs/ex_post_evaluation_en.pdf. Accessed 12 November 2019.

European Commission. (2011c). *Mid-term evaluation of the Health Strategy 2008–2013 Executive Summary*. Report prepared by "Public Health Evaluation and Impact Assessment Consortium" (PHEIAC). Accessed 21 March 2019.

European Commission. (2013a, September 23). *Reflection process: Innovative approaches for chronic diseases in public health and healthcare systems* [Note from the General Secretariat of the Council to Working Party on Public Health at Senior Level] Brussels. 12983/13. https://ec.europa.eu/health/sites/health/files/major_chronic_diseases/docs/reflection_process_cd_final_report_en.pdf. Accessed 12 November 2019.

European Commission. (2013b, August). *Evaluation of the use and impact of the European Community Health Indicators ECHI by Member States Executive summary*. https://ec.europa.eu/health/indicators/docs/echi_report_executive_summary_v20131031.pdf. Accessed 12 November 2019.

European Commission. (2013c). *Horizon 2020 budget* [factsheet]. https://ec.europa.eu/research/horizon2020/pdf/press/fact_sheet_on_horizon2020_budget.pdf. Accessed 13 November 2019.

European Commission. (2014a, April 4). *Communication from the Commission on effective, accessible and resilient health systems*. Brussels. COM(2014) 215 final. https://ec.europa.eu/health//sites/health/files/systems_performance_assessment/docs/com2014_215_final_en.pdf. Accessed 12 November 2019.

European Commission. (2014b). *Third EU Health Programme 2014–2020* [PowerPoint presentation]. https://ec.europa.eu/health/sites/health/files/programme/docs/ev_20141104_co01_en.pdf. Accessed 12 November 2019.

European Commission. (2014c). *The Third Health Programme 2014–2020 Funding Health Initiatives: The EU Health Programme in a Nutshell*. https://ec.europa.eu/health/sites/health/files/programme/docs/factsheet_healthprogramme2014_2020_en.pdf. Accessed 12 November 2019.

European Commission. (2014d, February 26). *Q&A on the third Health Programme 2014–2020* [Memo]. PDF download available from: https://ec.europa.eu/commission/presscorner/detail/en/MEMO_14_139. Accessed 12 November 2019.

European Commission. (2015a). *Ex-post Evaluation of the Health Programme (2008–2013)*. Final Report. https://ec.europa.eu/health/sites/health/files/programme/docs/ex-post_ev-hp-2008-13_final-report.pdf. Accessed 12 November 2019.

European Commission. (2015b). *Horizon 2020 Work Programme 2014–2015: 8. Health, demographic change and wellbeing – Revised*. Consolidated version following (European Commission Decision C (2015)2453 of 17 April. https://ec.europa.eu/research/participants/data/ref/h2020/wp/2014_2015/main/h2020-wp1415-health_en.pdf. Accesses 12 November 2019.

European Commission. (2016a, January 15). *Mapping of the use of European structural and investment funds in health in the 2007–2013 and 2014–2020 programming periods*. https://www.esifforhealth.eu/pdf/Mapping_Report_Final.pdf. Accessed 12 November 2019.

European Commission. (2016b). *Mandate of the Steering Group on Promotion and Prevention*. https://ec.europa.eu/health/sites/health/files/major_chronic_diseases/docs/sgpp_mandate_en.pdf. Accessed 12 November 2019.

European Commission. (2017a). State of Health in the EU: Companion Report 2017. https://ec.europa.eu/health/sites/health/files/state/docs/2017_companion_en.pdf. Accessed 12 November 2019.

European Commission. (2017b). *Better regulation 'toolbox'*. https://ec.europa.eu/info/sites/info/files/better-regulation-toolbox_2.pdf. Accessed 12 November 2019.

European Commission. (2017c). *European semester thematic factsheet: Health systems*. https://ec.europa.eu/info/sites/info/files/file_import/european-semester_thematic-factsheet_health-systems_en_0.pdf. Accessed 18 March 2019.

European Commission. (2017d, December 20). *Strategic Plan 2016–2020: DG health & food safety*. https://ec.europa.eu/info/sites/info/files/strategic-plan-2016-2020-dg-sante_en_0.pdf. Accessed 28 March 2019.

European Commission. (2017e). *Horizon 2020 Work Programme 2016–2017: 8. Health, demographic change and wellbeing* (European Commission Decision C(2017)2468 of 24 April 2017). https://ec.europa.eu/research/participants/data/ref/h2020/wp/2016_2017/main/h2020-wp1617-health_en.pdf. Accessed 12 November 2019.

European Commission. (2017f). *Country health profiles* [State of Health in the EU] [Website]. https://ec.europa.eu/health/state/country_profiles_en. Accessed 12 November 2019.

European Commission. (2017g). *Mid-term Evaluation of the third Health Programme (2014–2020) Final report*. https://ec.europa.eu/health/sites/health/files/programme/docs/2014-2020_evaluation_study_en.pdf. Accessed 12 November 2019.

European Commission. (2017h). *Personalised medicine: Focusing on citizen's health* [Infographic]. https://ec.europa.eu/research/health/pdf/personal-medicine_infographic_2018.pdf. Accessed 15 November 2019.

European Commission. (2018a, July 17). Commission decision setting up a Commission expert group "Steering Group on Health Promotion, Disease Prevention and Management of Non-Communicable Diseases" and repealing the Decision setting up a Commission expert group on rare diseases and the Decision establishing a Commission expert group on Cancer Control. https://ec.europa.eu/health/sites/health/files/major_chronic_diseases/docs/c2018_4492_en.pdf. Accessed 12 November 2019.

European Commission. (2018b, November 5). Mandate for a temporary subgroup on proton therapy centres [Steering Group on Health Promotion, Disease Prevention and Management of Non-Communicable Diseases]. https://ec.europa.eu/health/sites/health/files//non_communicable_diseases/docs/mandate_subgroup_protontherapycentres_en.pdf. Accessed 12 November 2019.

European Commission. (2018c, April 25). Commission Staff Working Document accompanying the document on enabling the digital transformation of health and care in the Digital Single Market; empowering citizens and building a healthier society [Communication From The Commission To The European Parliament, The Council, The European Economic And Social Committee and The Committee of the Regions] Brussels. SWD(2018) 126 final. PDF download available from: https://ec.europa.eu/digital-single-market/en/news/communication-enabling-digital-transformation-health-and-care-digital-single-market-empowering. Accessed 12 November 2019.

European Commission. (2018d). *Voluntary exchanges* [State of Health in the EU] [Webpage]. https://ec.europa.eu/health/state/voluntary_exchanges_en. Accessed 12 November 2019.

European Commission. (2018e). The Multiannual Financial Framework for 2021–2027: A Modern Budget for a Union that Protects, Empowers and Defends [Communication From The Commission To The European Parliament, The European Council, The Council, The European Economic And Social Committee And The Committee Of The Regions]. Brussels, 2 May. COM(2018) 321 final. https://eur-lex.europa.eu/resource.html?uri=cellar:c2bc7dbd-4fc3-11e8-be1d-01aa75ed71a1.0023.02/DOC_1&format=PDF. Accessed 12 November 2019.

European Commission. (2019a). *ESI Funds for Health: Investing for a healthy and inclusive EU. Final Report*. http://www.esifundsforhealth.eu/sites/default/files/2019-03/Final%20Report%20ESI%20Funds%20for%20Health_2.pdf. Accessed 12 November 2019.

European Commission. (2019b). Horizon 2020 Work Programme 2018–2020: 8. Health, demographic change and wellbeing. (European Commission Decision C(2019)4575 of 2 July). https://ec.europa.eu/research/participants/data/ref/h2020/wp/2018-2020/main/h2020-wp1820-health_en.pdf. Accessed 12 November 2019.

European Commission. (n.d.a). Criteria to Select Best Practices in Health Promotion and Chronic Disease Prevention and Management in Europe [Steering Group on Promotion and Prevention]. https://ec.europa.eu/health/sites/health/files/major_chronic_diseases/docs/sgpp_bestpracticescriteria_en.pdf. Accessed 12 November 2019.

European Commission. (n.d.b). *Overview* [State of Health in the EU] [Website]. https://ec.europa.eu/health/state/summary_en. Accessed 12 November 2019.

European Commission. (n.d.c). *Health at a Glance: Europe* [State of Health in the EU] [Website]. https://ec.europa.eu/health/state/glance_en. Accessed 12 November 2019.

European Commission. (n.d.d). *The European Core Health Indicators (ECHI) shortlist of 88 health indicators identified by policy area* [Appendix]. https://

ec.europa.eu/health/sites/health/files/indicators/docs/echi_shortlist_by_policy_area_en.pdf. Accessed 12 November 2019.

European Commission. (n.d.e). *Personalised Medicine: Background, conference reports, publications and links related to personalised medicine* [Website]. https://ec.europa.eu/research/health/index.cfm?pg=policy&policyname=personalised. Accessed 15 November 2019.

European Court of Auditors. (2009). The European Union's Public Health Programme (2003–07): An Effective Way to Improve Health? [Special Report No 2]. https://www.eca.europa.eu/lists/ecadocuments/sr09_02/sr09_02_en.pdf. Accessed 12 November 2019.

European Union. (2002, September 23). Decision No 1786/2002/Ec of the European Parliament and of the Council adopting a programme of Community action in the field of public health (2003–2008). *Official Journal of the European Communities*. https://eur-lex.europa.eu/resource.html?uri=cellar:7c8e9bce-dcf7-4bd8-9b94-e919bf5c6884.0004.02/DOC_1&format=PDF. Accessed 12 November 2019.

European Union. (2014, March 11). Regulation (EU) no 282/2014 of the European Parliament and of the Council on the establishment of a third Programme for the Union's action in the field of health (2014–2020) and repealing Decision No 1350/2007/EC. *Official Journal of the European Union*. https://eur-lex.europa.eu/legal-content/EN/TXT/PDF/?uri=CELEX:32014R0282&from=EN. Accessed 12 November 2019.

Fairclough, N. (2003). *Analysing discourse: Textual analysis for social research*. Routledge.

Ferlie, E., & McGivern, G. (2014). Bringing anglo-governmentality into public management scholarship: The case of evidence-based medicine in UK health care. *Journal of Public Administration Research and Theory, 24*(1), 59–83.

Flear, M. (2015). *Governing public health: EU law, regulation and biopolitics*. Hart Publishing.

Glasgow, S., & Schrecker, T. (2016). The double burden of neoliberalism? Noncommunicable disease policies and the global political economy of risk. *Health and Place, 39*, 204–211.

Goodwin, P., & Wright, G. (2004). *Decision analysis for management judgement* (3rd ed.). Wiley.

Greenhalgh, T., & Russell, J. (2009). Evidence-based policymaking: A critique. *Perspectives in Biology and Medicine, 52*(2), 304–318.

Greer, S. L., Fahy, N., Heather, A. E., Wismar, M., Jarman, H., Palm, W., Elliott, H. A., & Wismar, M. (2014). *Everything you always wanted to know about European Union health policies but were too afraid to ask*. The European Observatory on Health Systems and Policies. Tetragon.

Jamison, D., Yamey, G., Beyeler, N., & Wadge, H. (2016). Investing in health: The economic case. *World Innovation Summit for Health* [Doha, Qatar].

Karanikolos, M., Mladovsky, P., Cylus, J., Thomson, S., Basu, S., Stuckler, D., Mackenbach, J. P., McKee, M. (2013). Financial crisis, austerity, and health in Europe. *The Lancet, 381*(9874), 1323–1331.

Kentikelenis, A., Karanikolos, M., Papanicolas, I., Basu, S., McKee, M., et al. (2011). Health effects of financial crisis: Omens of a Greek tragedy. *The Lancet, 378*(9801), 1457–1458.

Kickbusch, I. (1989). Approaches to an ecological base for public health. *Health Promotion, 4*(4), 265–268.

Koivusalo, M. (2010). The State of Health in All Policies (HiAP) in the European Union: Potential and pitfalls. *Journal of Epidemiology and Community Health, 64*(6), 500–503.

Lane, J. E. (2000). *New public management*. Routledge.

Lynch, J. (2020). *Regimes of inequality—The political economy of health and wealth*. Cambridge University Press.

McInnes, C. (2015). The many meanings of health security. In S. Rushton & J. Youde (Eds.), *Routledge handbook of global health security* (pp. 7–17). Routledge.

Marston, G., & Watts, R. (2003). Tampering with the evidence a critical appraisal of evidence-based policy-making. *The Drawing Board: an Australian Review of Public Affairs, 3*(3), 143–163.

McKee, M., Reeves, A., Clair, A., & Stuckler, D. (2017). Living on the edge: Precariousness and why it matters for health. *Archives of Public Health, 75*(13). https://doi.org/10.1186/s13690-017-0183-y

McKenna, B., & Graham, P. (2000). Technocratic discourse: A primer. *Journal of Technical Writing and Communication, 30*(3), 223–251.

McLaren, L., McIntyre, L., & Kirkpatrick, S. (2010). Rose's population strategy of prevention need not increase social inequalities in health. *International Journal of Epidemiology, 39*(2), 372–377.

Neylan, J. (2008). Social policy and the authority of evidence. *The Australian Journal of Public Administration, 67*(1), 12–19.

Nutley, S., Powell, A., & Davies, H. (2013). What counts as good evidence? Provocation paper for the alliance for useful evidence. Research Unit for Research Utilisation. School of Management, University of St. Andrews. https://www.alliance4usefulevidence.org/assets/What-Counts-as-Good-Evidence-WEB.pdf. Accessed 11 November 2019.

OECD. (2010). *Health care systems: Getting more value for money* (Economics department policy notes, No. 2).

Parkhurst, J., & Abeysinghe, S. (2016). What constitutes "good" evidence for public health and social policy-making? From Hierarchies to Appropriateness. *Social Epistemology, 30*(5–6), 665–679.

Parkhurst, J. (2017). *The politics of evidence: From evidence-based policy to the good governance of evidence*. Routledge.

Petticrew, M., & Roberts, H. (2003). Evidence, hierarchies, and typologies: Horses for courses. *Journal of Epidemiology and Community Health, 57*, 527–529.

Petticrew, M., Katikireddi, S. V., Knai, C., Cassidy, R., Maani Hessari, N., Thomas, J., & Weishaar, H. (2017). 'Nothing can be done until everything is done': The use of complexity arguments by food, beverage, alcohol and gambling industries. *Journal of Epidemiology and Community Health, 71*(11), 1078–1083.

Purser, R. E., Forbes, D., & Burke, A. (Eds.). (2016). *Handbook of mindfulness: Culture, context, and social engagement* [eBook]: Springer.

Ronit, K., & Jensen, J. D. (2014). Obesity and industry self-regulation of food and beverage marketing: A literature review. *European Journal of Clinical Nutrition, 68*(7), 753–759.

Rose, G. (1985). Sick individuals and sick populations. *International Journal of Epidemiology, 14*(1), 32–38.

Rushton, S., & Williams, O. D. (2012). Frames, Paradigms and power: Global health policy-making under neoliberalism. *Global Society, 26*(2), 147–167.

Sachs, J. (2001). *Macroeconomics and health: Investing in health for economic development*. Report of the Commission on Macroeconomics and Health. Geneva: World Health Organization.

Sanderson, I. (2006). Complexity, 'practical rationality' and evidence based policy making. *Policy & Politics, 34*(1), 115–132.

Savona, N., Thompson, C., Smith, D., & Cummins, S. (2020). 'Complexity' as a rhetorical smokescreen for UK public health inaction on diet. *Critical Public Health*. https://doi.org/10.1080/09581596.2020.1755421

Singh, G. K., & Siapush, M. (2006). Widening socioeconomic inequalities in US life expectancy, 1980–2000. *International Journal of Epidemiology, 35*(4), 969–979.

Smith, K. E. (2013). *Beyond evidence-based policy in public health: The interplay of ideas*. Palgrave Macmillan.

Smith, K. E. (2014). The politics of ideas: The complex interplay of health inequalities research and policy. *Science and Public Policy, 41*(5), 561–574.

Smith, K. E., & Joyce, K. E. (2012). Capturing complex realities: understanding efforts to achieve evidence-based policy and practice in public health. *Evidence & Policy, 8*(1), 57–78.

Ståhl, T., Wismar, M., Ollila, E., Lahtinen, E., & Leppo, K. (Eds.). (2006). *Health in All Policies: Prospects and potentials*. Ministry of Social Affairs and Health, Finland.

Stuckler, D., Reeves, A., Loopstra, R., Karanikolos, M., & McKee, M. (2017). Austerity and health: The impact in the UK and Europe. *European Journal of Public Health, 27*(Suppl. 4), 18–21.

Weiss, C. H. (1977). Research for policy's sake: The enlightenment function of social research. *Policy Analysis, 3*(4), 531–545.

Weiss, C. H. (1979). The many meanings of research utilization. *Public Administration Review, 39*(5), 426–431.

Wilkinson, R. G., & Pickett, K. (2010). *The spirit level: Why equality is better for everyone* (2nd ed.). Penguin Books.

CHAPTER 7

Shifting Focus: Why Did 'Health in All Policies' Still Reach the EU?

This chapter examines the politics of defining HiAP. It explores why HiAP was successful in reaching the EU space, but also why it is prone to being watered down and co-opted. I argue that this is because HiAP is a chameleonic idea (Smith, 2013a). That means it is strategically phrased to appeal to the people it seeks to reach (EU policymakers). Chameleonic ideas maintain an intentional level of vagueness, and their meaning is therefore easy to change, to recycle or to co-opt. The analysis in this chapter shows how the chameleonic nature of HiAP explains its success in reaching the EU space. However, once in the EU space, the meaning of HiAP evolves in ways that are difficult to control, which adds to why HiAP did not lead to radical changes. This chapter identifies several ways in which HiAP becomes actively redefined in a way that promotes institutional continuity and that does not address macrosocial determinants of health. I then explore how ideas like HiAP also become recycled in renewed attempts to induce change and counter co-option, and I argue that the 'wellbeing economy' theme of the 2019 Finnish EU presidency is example of such recycling of ideas.

After having explored the prevailing structural obstacles to a more meaningful HiAP uptake, this last chapter turns the focus towards HiAP itself, and the nature of this idea, its meaning. If the EU is institutionally and ideationally incompatible with HiAP, how is it that the idea still

C. Godziewski, *The Politics of Health Promotion*,
Palgrave Studies in Science, Knowledge and Policy,
https://doi.org/10.1007/978-3-030-97870-9_7

became officially endorsed by the European Commission and the Council (EU Council, 2006a; European Commission, 2007a)? Was it all rhetoric, or did HiAP still manage to induce some change?

To explore these questions, we move to DI's third element: foreground discursive abilities. We will locate agency in power *through* ideas (the power of agents to convince of the validity of an idea), as well as power *over* idea (the capacity of agents to define, redefine and shape what ideas mean, what defines them). To do so, the chapter will draw on Smith's (2013a) concept of 'chameleonic ideas'. Her categorisation of ideas includes a chameleonic type, which refers to ideas *strategically* formulated to become accepted in spaces where incompatible institutional set ups and background ideational structures prevail. The 'strategic' formulation here is key, as it points to the agential, foreground discursive space in which agents can articulate discourses that are critical of their institutions, and do so in a way which they perceive will maximise the potential for endogenous institutional change. Empirically, this analysis is heavily informed by interview data gathered in Helsinki and Tampere, during the second round of interviews and with people involved in promoting the HiAP agenda in the EU. In order to analyse the power dynamics around the meaning of HiAP prevailing in the EU, and visible in the language used around HiAP in EU documents, it draws on the insights provided by the Finnish interviewees, as well as by EU health advocates, regarding the strategies used to get HiAP accepted in the EU, as well as their insights regarding the dangers of co-option.

The following sections will explore some of the ways in which the meaning of HiAP is negotiated and redefined. It then delves into the implications of the chameleonic nature of HiAP: that its meaning is a constant and ever-evolving political battleground. First, it looks at discursive efforts to maintain institutional continuity. This includes redefinitions of HiAP as inherently about multistakeholder involvement, as well as the use of HiAP language to promote EC priority streamlining more generally. Both these discursive adaptations in HiAP meaning represent attempts to fit HiAP into a technocratic NMG context. While the extent to which these particular dynamics are the result of structure, agency or a mix of both, is impossible to tell, the chapter does point to elements that emphasise the agential role of individuals, including EU officials and industry lobbyists (for EU food and drink industry lobby tactics, see for example: Tselengidis & Östergren, 2019). The risk of HiAP being a chameleonic idea and which is pointed out in these parts of the chapter, is that because it is couched in dominant EU language and because of its intentional normative ambiguity, it can become (easily) co-opted and watered down.

However, this does not mean that HiAP advocates (who advocate for HiAP on a normative ground) are unaware of these shifts. The second half of the chapter analyses documents related to the most recent (2019) Finnish EU presidency and looks at how foreground discursive abilities have been mobilised to reshape the fluid, vague and chameleonic idea that is HiAP into new versions of itself, in order to continue to promote endogenous institutional change. In the same way that HiAP is a development from the Health for All agenda from the 1970s, HiAP can be further modified, rethought and rearticulated in ways that seek to address the risks of co-option in the EU institutional setting (Smith, 2013b). I suggest that the 2019 Finnish EU presidency theme 'economy of wellbeing' can be thought as an evolution of HiAP. Furthermore, the newly created advocacy coalition that promotes a health-centred economy of wellbeing, the 'All Policies for a Healthy Europe' initiative, aims to shape that concept in a way that seeks to address pitfalls faced by HiAP. The figure below provides an overview of the tensions and different directions in which the meaning of HiAP evolves: either towards institutional continuity or towards a recycled version of itself.

Finally, the last section of this chapter explores the potential for synergies between chameleonic ideas like HiAP and more radical ones like degrowth. Indeed, with the shift from HiAP to economy of wellbeing, and from health to wellbeing, a greater accent has been put on the critique of gross domestic product (GDP). While the EU's position on economy of wellbeing does not challenge the economic growth paradigm (it only proposes that growth should be 'smart, sustainable and inclusive' without necessarily too much explanation of what this means concretely), the degrowth (or post-growth) idea is more radical in taking the critique of GDP further, to posit that growth itself is a problem (or 'the' problem). Surprisingly, even a radical idea like degrowth can be found in the EU institutions, albeit in a very limited number of places. Degrowth is nevertheless put forward by individuals from the JRC and from the EP. Figure 7.1 provides an overview of this chapter's rationale and argument.

While it is important to recognise the space for agency and contestation, we need to remain cautious and not overly naïve about the potential for an idea like HiAP to bring about any kind of radical change. Instead, the imaginable change that HiAP-like ideas could bring about

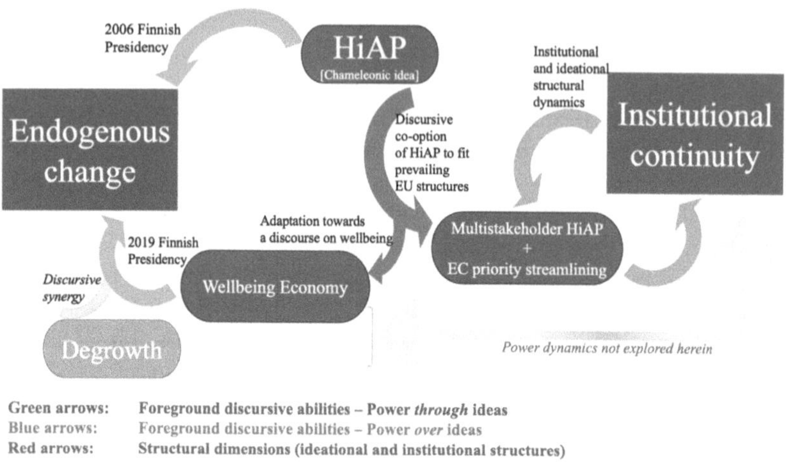

Fig. 7.1 Chapter overview: exploring foreground discursive abilities around HiAP

relates more to an endogenous, gradual and slow process of evolution than a radical game-changer. Determining whether this is the best—or a successful—strategy is not the aim here. What this analysis suggests, is that for chameleonic ideas like HiAP to avoid being watered down and forgotten, they require constant recycling and re-invention.

7.1 Chameleonic Ideas and Endogenous Institutional Change

Schmidt's DI argues for the need to look at the role of ideas to understand and explain institutional change and continuity. The level of ideational power looked at in this chapter is the level of foreground, discursively articulated idea definition, the power *over* and *through* ideas. In the vein of focusing on ideas, Smith (2013a) has argued that analysing evidence without ideational and discursive context is insufficient to understand health policymaking. She argues that, to better understand health policy, one needs to look beyond research evidence and instead investigate the importance of ideas in shaping, enabling or constraining health policies, importance which arguably exceeds the role of research evidence 'alone'. She identifies four types of ideas: institutional ideas, which do not aim to challenge the status quo. Radical ideas, which are too radical to become widely adopted in the policymaking sphere. Research that talks explicitly about *neoliberalism* and health tends to fit into this category. Charismatic ideas are very rare and represent radical ideas that have 'made it' and have become commonly accepted, without compromising their radical essence. Among those kinds of ideas and in relation to health policy, Smith (2013a) takes the example of tobacco legislation, and how health promotion related to tobacco reduction is now largely dealt with hard laws and regulations, unlike much of the rest of 'lifestyle-related' health promotion confined to voluntary, soft governance.

Finally, chameleonic ideas are ideas that may have a normative essence, and may have originally been put forward to try to change the status quo, but that have been strategically adapted, and are sufficiently vague, in order to become institutionally accepted. One characteristic of chameleonic ideas is their appeal to normative neutrality. The normative nature of these ideas is intentionally toned down to fit the language of the policymaking sphere, and the idea is vague enough to strategically allow room for interpretation. Similarly, Smith (2010, 2012, 2014) describes how the language of chameleonic ideas is adjusted to fit the academic funding bodies' language, in order to increase the chance for research to receive funding. Chameleonic ideas also result from academic peer pressures exercised in different directions: on the one hand, academics who are perceived as too close to policymakers can be subject to criticism for their perceived lack of independence. On the other hand, arguments put forward by academics who are perceived as too ideological can be dismissed by some peers on the basis that they are 'too biased'.

> [...]some academics described presenting their work to policy audiences (who were perceived as both potential research users and, importantly, potential funders) in ways that emphasised the aspects of their work that they felt were most likely to be received favourably and/or deliberately imbuing challenging ideas with chameleon-like qualities to ensure that they were not deemed 'too radical'. (Smith & Joyce, 2012, p. 66)

These are some of the tensions to navigate in the context of academics working on health inequalities, but these tensions also apply for advocates and researchers of HiAP: the challenge is to find a way to put forward a normatively driven idea that changes the status quo, without being perceived as too ideological and losing credibility from policymakers and potentially even from peers and funders (Smith, 2010, 2012, 2014).

The ramifications of Smith's argument (2010, 2012, 2014) around researchers needing to appear neutral and serious in order to get funding and in order to get their ideas heard point to the complex relationship and power dynamics between academic research and health policymaking. They also point to the dominance of the instrumental view of the relationship between research and policymaking (Weiss, 1977, 1979), a dominance which public health scholarship contributes to building. To address the pitfalls of the dominance of instrumental relationships between policy and research, Mykhalovskiy et al. (2019) call for more dialogue between 'social science *in* public health' and 'social science *of* public health'. The former refers to the largely positivist literature that is embedded in an institutional setting of natural science, medical public health research. They include academic researchers who work very closely with policymakers and aim to see their work leading to real-life results, pragmatically setting aside 'meta-critiques' of the system within which their expertise operates and focusing on (smaller) immediate improvements (Smith, 2012). The 'social science *of* public health' literature is embedded in social sciences, social health research, and includes critical social science approaches to public health, such as post-structuralist, Marxist or critical feminist frameworks. This group is made up of academics who focus on 'the big picture', on working towards changing society more fundamentally, but who often struggle to achieve tangible results. They would be the ones putting forward radical ideas, and theirs would be the work dismissed in the policymaking sphere as 'too ideological'.

What Mykhalovskiy et al. (2019) then suggest, is the creation of more space for agonistic engagement between critical social science and public health: 'critical social science *with* public health'. This would be a kind of critical social science literature that would combine both worlds without merging them, not compromising on its critical stance but at the same time being useful to public health practitioners. However, it could be argued that this space already exists, and that is occupied by those researchers putting forward chameleonic ideas. This kind of researcher, which Smith (2012) refers to as 'flexians', has already been grappling with the tensions between policy relevance and normativity. Flexians seek to negotiate these tensions by putting forward chameleonic ideas, being aware of the risk of appearing too ideological, while at the same time identifying the need to challenge the status quo deeply and fundamentally.

Power Through Ideas: Chameleonic HiAP

An idea being chameleonic does not mean that researchers advocating for it are unaware of the normative implications or are not driven by those norms. The question then becomes about the merits of radical ideas in research, that do not compromise on their normativity but run the risk of not being heard where they should be heard, and the merits of chameleonic ideas in research, which strategically tone down their normativity in order to reach the policymaking spheres, but which then run the risk of becoming appropriated, reshaped and lose their normative essence. Is it more useful to outright reject the economic paradigm of health, or to try to channel it towards a more HiAP-like vision? Answering this question is beyond the scope of this book. However, it can be argued that, while radical ideas aim for exogenous, revolutionary change, chameleonic ideas seek endogenous, evolutionary change. To put it in relation to HiAP, inequities and macrosocial determinants of health, chameleonic ideas seek to ease into the notion that neoliberal policies are detrimental to health by highlighting effects of neoliberal governance, rather than confront and name that system outright. In her book, Lynch (2020) talks about these kinds of trade-offs and argues that talking about 'health inequalities' is problematic because the medicalisation of social problems reinforces the notion that certain political ideas—redistribution, regulation, public spending—have become decidedly unacceptable, even taboo. From this perspective, well-intentioned chameleonic strategies do more harm than good (especially on the long term), because they internalise these taboos rather than challenging them.

Nevertheless, an important aspect of chameleonic ideas is the notion of intentionality, of agency. Chameleonic ideas are *strategically* articulated, and while they do run the risk of becoming co-opted and watered down, those putting forward chameleonic ideas for health policy tend to be well aware of those risks and attempt to actively and critically navigate them. As such, the use of chameleonic ideas can be conceptualised in terms of 'foreground discursive ability', of space for agents to articulate a discourse critical of their institution, or, on the contrary, to actively shape ideas to suit the overarching institutional and ideational context. The purpose of this chapter is then to identify and reflect upon different ways in which HiAP is talked about, by whom, and to assess what is being actively discursively done with HiAP (the 'politics of defining HiAP' [Koivusalo, 2019]).

Strategies to Propose HiAP at EU Level

As a chameleonic idea, HiAP is adapted to EU language, and its normative essence is acknowledged only to the extent that it remains perceived as reasonable, not too 'ideological'. At the time of the Finnish 2006 presidency, the explicitness of the normativity of HiAP and public health more generally had to be negotiated. HiAP, from the perspective of the Finnish health policymakers and researchers interviewed, was very clearly a translation from the Ottawa Charter's health promotion strategy to fit the EU, and to operationalise the EU Treaty language on protecting health in all policies. However, according to two interviewees who participated in the 2006 Finnish presidency agenda setting, negotiating the commitment to public health-related norms in the EU Council demanded discursive strategising. For example, instead of taking a radical stance which might have led to rejection, they presented the norms underpinning EU health systems as already commonly accepted and already shared:

> The story of how the [Council] conclusions[1] put the stress on common values: In negotiating that, they got into problems when they tried to say that everybody should have equity and equality and so on, as a value. And somehow, they got into problems at the high-level commission for health. But then the great idea of one of the people in charge was to present those values not as 'we need to impose them' but present them as 'these are the values that we already have'. So, you avoid those problems. (Quoted from interviewee 31)

The strategy for introducing the emphasis on shared values is very interesting, because it shows how the Finnish team understood the need to avoid appearing overly ideological, and that the way to do it was to assert the value in question as a taken-for-granted assumption. This may have represented a powerful defence against the commonly held critique that HiAP is 'health imperialistic' (see Kemm, 2001; Synnevåg et al., 2018). Additionally, they put the accent on Article 168, and the notion that HiAP is in fact nothing inherently new and radical, but merely a *return* to taking Article 168 more seriously. The strong normativity of HiAP was to an extent 'toned down' and made palatable to the EU (and member states) policymaking crowd, both in terms of making a strong treaty basis

[1] The conclusions referred to by the interviewee are the 2006 Council Conclusions on Common values and principles in European Union Health Systems (EU Council, 2006b).

case (Art. 168 TFEU), as well as in terms of constructing a language of normative reasonableness compatible with the EU institutional setting.

This instance of intentionally using the discursive malleability of HiAP already points to the foreground discursive capacities of the 2006 Finnish Presidency team members that allowed HiAP to even be introduced into the EU space in the first place. It represents an instance of power *through* ideas. Indeed, those individuals were acting within their own national and European overlapping institutional boundaries, and yet were able to put forward an idea that, at its core, challenges EU orthodoxy, and to make it accepted within those institutions. Arguably, and based on interviewee's insights,[2] the HLG still represents a space of broadly like-minded health experts in which HiAP strategising can take place, even though the capacity of the group to bring about fundamental change is limited.

The power struggles over the meaning of HiAP, however, do not stop here. The next section analyses how some agents 'used their foreground discursive abilities' to shape or 'change the contours' (Smith, 2013b, p. 82) of HiAP in a way that fits the prevailing EU (neoliberal) orthodoxy.

7.2 Institutionalised HiAP

If an idea is vague enough to be either fitted to the language dominating in a particular institutional context or to contest the institution, then whatever happens to the idea after it has been introduced can be difficult to predict, and becomes a site of power struggle. Institutional context and ideational abilities, as seen in previous chapters, will inevitably have an impact on how the idea changes and evolves. But it also depends on intentional, 'agential' discourse articulation around that idea. This section explores how foreground discursive abilities have been mobilised to shape the meaning of HiAP in a way that suits the prevailing EU institutional orthodoxy, effectively the 'watering down' forces. It explores how HiAP is being made to fit the NMG rationale, both by being made to be about multistakeholder engagement and by being used to justify streamlining EU economic priorities. Of course, it is never entirely possible to disentangle the structural from the agential dynamics. In turn, some phenomena can be explained both in terms of structural and agential

[2] Source: interviewees 15, 17, 18, 19, and 27.

power dynamics.[3] Nevertheless, this section draws on interview material to make sense of some of the *active* and suggested *intentional*, discursive strategising around HiAP, and how it is being made to fit existing priorities, in other words, how it risks becoming watered down.

Multistakeholder HiAP

One of the characteristics attributed to HiAP in some settings, including the EU, is that it is inherently about involving all the stakeholders. In the main documents prepared by Finland on HiAP in 2006, there is limited mention of engagement with private stakeholders (except most notably in chapters three and five in Ståhl et al., 2006). And while these chapters do encourage multistakeholder engagement to some extent, they remain cautious and emphasise the risk of conflict of interest (Ståhl et al., 2006). The 2006 policy brief does not refer to private sector engagement as an important component of HiAP at all (Ollila et al., 2006). However, the subsequent EU documents contain several mentions of the importance of involving all stakeholders (EU Council, 2006a; European Commission, 2007a). The boxes below highlight some of those instances:

Box 7.1 Council Conclusions on Health in All Policies (HiAP) (EU Council, 2006a, p. 7)
The Council of the European Union [...]

INVITES the Commission [...]

to encourage and support exchange of good practices and information on intersectoral policies between Community sectors, Member States, and other stakeholders [...]

INVITES the Member States [...]

take into account in the formulation and implementation of their national policies the added value offered by cooperation between government sector, social partners, the private sector, and the non-governmental organisations for public health.

[3] In this book, this is the case for the phenomenon of increased involvement of the European Semester in health: it has already been looked at from an institutional and ideational structural perspective, and this chapter will shed light onto the agential dimensions of that phenomenon.

Box 7.2 White Paper—Together for Health: A Strategic Approach for the EU 2008–2013 (European Commission, 2007a, p. 6)
[...] HIAP is also about involving new partners in health policy. The Commission will develop partnerships to promote goals of the Strategy, including with NGOs, industry, academia and the media [...].

It is impossible to ascertain whether this change in meaning of HiAP—this instance of 'power *over* idea'—is purely the result of structures described previously, or of discursive agency, or to what extent it results from a blend of both. This is where the non-binary, co-constitutive nature of the structure/agency 'scale' is most visible, and it would be naïve to think of those individuals who have interpreted HiAP as inherently multistakeholder, as people acting obliviously and purely under the subconscious effect of ideational and institutional structures. Events that end up being pivotal in how HiAP is defined can be mundane and contingent. For example, in the context of HiAP in Finland, the disappointing outcomes of the 2014 meetings on a national HiAP strategy (see Chapter 2) were, according to the interviewee,[4] in large part down to the agency of a few individuals in specific positions at that particular time.

It is also possible to identify some specific points of discursive constructions of multistakeholder HiAP: one concrete path through which this addition to the meaning of HiAP can be made visible is the ambiguity of the term 'sector'. Indeed, 'intersectoral', including in relation to action for health, was originally meant to refer to collaboration across public sectors, i.e. the different public policy areas within governments.[5] Applied to the EC governance, this would refer to collaboration across DGs only. However more recently, 'intersectoral' has been used to refer to different sectors of society, i.e. the public, private and voluntary sectors (Ståhl et al., 2006, p. 5). Echoing the research done by Smith et al. (2015) which highlight the active role of the tobacco industry in shaping the EU regulatory landscape, it is reasonable to suspect that individuals representing industries related to NCDs (such as, for example, tobacco, food and soft drinks and alcohol) have an interest in actively shaping HiAP as inherently multistakeholder in order to secure a seat at the table and be able to

[4] Source: interviewee 31.

[5] Source: interviewee 32.

shape the HiAP implementation process in ways which do not threaten their interests (see also the point made by Tselengidis & Östergren [2019, p. 572] regarding 'constituency building' as a lobby strategy used by the EU food and drink industry).

Importantly though, according to key Finnish experts involved in setting up the EU HiAP agenda in 2006, HiAP was never meant to refer to the involvement of all sectors of society. It was instead meant to refer to the involvement and prioritisation of health in all sectors of government.[6]

> In Finland there's consultation with private sector and NGOs in the beginning, in the end, but not throughout! Importantly, the HiAP concept never intended to mean 'multistakeholder' and PPPs [private-public partnerships], 'intersectoral' refers to the different public, government sectors, but not to private/public/non-profit sectors. That's something that was misinterpreted. (Quoted from interviewee 32)

The same idea was suggested already in 2010 (Koivusalo, 2010, p. 500): 'The main essence of the approach implicitly implies that the focus is on *public policies* and activities across different "policies", not, for example, between public and private sector' (emphasis in original text). The conflation of HiAP as multistakholder is problematic because it implies that the responsibility for HiAP is diffused towards other sectors of society. As such, it represents an avenue for lifestyle drift and all the problems associated with it (see Chapter 5). Ultimately 'multistakeholder HiAP' reflects an alignment of HiAP with some of the main NMG tenets around blurring the line between private and public sector. The awareness of Finnish HiAP advocates of the consequences of the multistakeholder interpretation of HiAP, shows that HiAP proponents are driven by a normative vision that is *strategically* toned down. And while one Finnish interviewee[7] regretted that they had not defined HiAP more clearly at the time (to avoid the multistakeholder interpretation), this chapter suggests that defining it much more clearly might have jeopardised its very uptake at EU level, if it had meant straightforward normative explicitness, i.e. HiAP might no longer have been a chameleonic idea, but a radical one.

[6] Source: interviewees 31 and 32.

[7] Source: interviewees 32.

HiAP as Streamlining EC Priorities

This section looks at how HiAP language and references to mainstreaming have, prior to the pandemic, been used in the proposal to integrate the health programme into a wider European Social Fund+ (ESF+) in the upcoming MFF, considering the ESF+ 's ever-closer ties to the European Semester process. It suggests that, while HiAP initially was used to refer to the need for other sectors to work towards health, explicitly including the EC itself, there may be a risk of now mentioning HiAP in a broader sense of 'there needs to be an EC coherence, less silo thinking and therefore a better alignment of SANTE to EC priorities'. In other words, HiAP risks becoming amalgamated with (and subordinated to) a more general discourse of needing to streamline priorities, create synergies and move beyond silo-thinking. But in the process, the notion that *health* is what needs to be mainstreamed gets lost, and instead the search for coherence revolves around typical EU priorities: growth, competitiveness and fiscal discipline. While acknowledging the institutional and ideational dynamics explored in the previous chapters and which facilitate this kind of drift, this chapter touches upon the possible role of individual agents in this process.

The empirical example used here is a historical analysis of the negotiations of the 2021–2027 MFF, and the role of health within it, *prior to the outbreak of the pandemic*. It is very important to note that, after the pandemic broke out, there was a radical change in the place and resources attributed to health. Of course, the pandemic represents a shock to the system which is leading to rethinking the place of public health in EU governance. As this chapter draws on data collected between March 2018 and April 2019, it does not consider the impact of the COVID-19 pandemic on the MFF negotiations. As such, this empirical snapshot is no longer up to date. Nevertheless, this pre-COVID empirical experience provides useful and still relevant insights into the dynamics of streamlining EU priorities and how this can impact competing agendas. For example, at the time of writing, the EC has made available to member states grants and loans from the Recovery and Resilience Facility (RRF), a fund set up under the 'NextGenerationEU' instrument and specially aimed at mitigating the impact of the pandemic, as well as assist member states on their path to a greener, more digital economy (aligned with the European Green Deal priorities). In practice, a similar logic applies to the RRF as to the European Semester, with the same kinds of conditions and expectations attached to the member state's plans (European Commission, n.d.a).

Prior to the pandemic, the state of the MFF for 2021–2027 suggested that there should be no stand-alone health programme anymore, but that instead a separate health stream would be part of the new ESF, the 'ESF+' (European Commission, 2018a). The dedicated health budget within the ESIF has always been much larger than the modest stand-alone health programme. Nevertheless, the move to integrate the (former) health programme, along with other funds, within the ESF+ illustrated a stronger emphasis on streamlining priorities, merging programmes, shifting from a landscape of multiple fragmented programmes towards an integrated project. This was justified in terms of coherence, synergies and a strong emphasis on avoiding duplication. One interviewee from the EC explained that streamlining works to improve resource allocation, as it allows money to move around with greater flexibility.[8] The streamlining of health into the ESF+ was justified using the language and rationale of HiAP:

> Bridging the gap that separates health from non-health sectors is important for meaningful health outcomes from the European Structural and Investment Funds. [...] the inclusion of the EU Health Programme within an expanded ESF+ programme targeting implementation of the European Pillar of Social Rights (EPSR), should foster increased cross-sectoral collaboration at the strategic level. (European Commission, 2019a, p. 9)

The EC, through its plan to streamline health within the ESF+ , also aimed to deepen its involvement in member states' healthcare reforms, through the means of the European Semester. This reflected an awareness that policy areas are interconnected, yet it also suggested that health systems needed to be reformed through the lens of the EU's economic and fiscal governance, rather than thinking about how economic governance could be reformed so as to work towards health and wellbeing. Given its embeddedness in the ESF+, the EC's health activities were likely to be even more closely coordinated by the European Semester:

[8] Source: interviewee 28.

> The European Social Fund+ will be more closely aligned with the European Semester of economic policy coordination, which takes regional specificities into account. The detailed analysis of member states' challenges in the context of the European Semester will serve as a basis for the programming of the funds at the start and at mid-term of the next period. This will serve as the roadmap for the short, mid- and long-term planning and monitoring of the funds. A system of ex-ante conditionalities and macro-economic conditionality will be maintained. (European Commission, 2018b, p. 42)

Theoretically, the streamlining of the health programme in the broader social agenda has been seen as an opportunity, notably for HiAP, as it could have the potential to expand the consideration of health impacts of other policy areas. In fact, worth noting is the renewed emphasis that is currently being put on making the European Semester about wellbeing and sustainability, in the context of the new Commission's European Green Deal (European Commission, 2019b). However, some interviewees[9] were mostly raising the more pragmatic concern that horizontal integration may come at the detriment of protecting institutional safeguards. This concern needs to be considered in light of the institutional and ideational power dynamics explored in previous chapters, which already suggest a push towards neoliberalisation. Horizontal integration accompanied by a weakening of health in its own right could lead to a dilution of public health concerns. In other words, these interviewees were concerned that HiAP has been serving as a rhetorical tool to gradually water down actions in the field of public health. Some of the NGO interviewees feared that referring to HiAP will end up leading to installing one health desk in each DG, but without any coordinated, purposeful health plan.[10] This threat was perceived as especially salient given the general feeling among some NGO (and industry) interviewees,[11] that DG SANTE was gradually being side-lined. These concerns were not only present among NGO representatives, as indeed other interviewees from

[9] Source: interviewees 12, 13, 24 and 26.

[10] Source: interviewees 12 and 26.

[11] Source: interviewees 6, 12, 13, 21 and 26.

EU institutions and member states did stress the importance of institutional safeguards needed to counter potential dilution resulting from evermore horizontal integration and streamlining.[12]

Amplifying the concern regarding the risk of watering down HiAP, is the notion that individuals within big institutions like the EC, may not necessarily be driven by a passion for the particular branch they currently work in. While many individuals working for DG SANTE have health-specific qualifications and have dedicated their careers to public health (as was very much the case for Juncker's health commissioner, for example), others might have other backgrounds and other aspirations. One example of this pertains to one former DG SANTE Director General. When speaking at a press event about trans fatty acid regulation in April 2018, the then DG SANTE Director General's first point mentioned, before highlighting anything about health, was whether the industry was ready to accept regulation (Jennings, 2018). This was vehemently criticised by health advocates for betraying the lack of genuine concern for public health as the central aim of SANTE, and was taken by those health advocates as a Freudian slip confirming the sentiment they had already been developing: that this Director General was not particularly driven by a concern for public health. The main point here is not to single out and criticise individual members of DG SANTE, but rather, to put the emphasis on the existence of space for agency of individual SANTE officials.

One discursive pathway through which the amalgamation between HiAP and EU priorities streamlining can occur is the ambiguity of what the word 'mainstreaming' refers to. Differences in uses of the word mainstreaming, and their effect, have been emphasised in the context of EU gender mainstreaming, and this also apply in the context of HiAP and health mainstreaming:

> The word mainstreaming itself is subject to several interpretations. The term covers multiple meanings and contents, which have been used to conform Community gender policies to the competitiveness principle at work in European employment policies. (Bruno et al., 2006, p. 531)

Indeed, the notion of 'mainstreaming' can invoke a sense of deep embeddedness in a 'way of working'. This is the case notably for the Better

[12] Source: interviewees 8 and 27.

Regulation concept. Mainstreaming in the context of Better Regulation is used to convey a vision, a concept with 'a spirit' to follow.[13] Better Regulation has been described as being part of the EC 'DNA' (European Commission, 2017a, p. 2), and its scope is defined with much freedom:

> The Better Regulation Guidelines should be applied flexibly and in a proportionate manner that reflects the circumstances of each individual initiative. What matters is that *the spirit* of the Guidelines (and tools) is applied and that high quality IAs, evaluations etc. result. (European Commission, 2017b, p. 8 [emphasis added])

On the other hand, 'mainstreaming' can also be used to refer to a technocratic NMG tool which buys into, rather than challenges, neoliberalism (Bacchi & Eveline, 2010). Bruno et al. (2006) traced the origins of the concept of gender mainstreaming in the EU back to the 1980s. They then identified a change in the use of the word mainstreaming in around 1995, when a group of individuals not immediately tied to gender-related work defined it in terms of an NMG tool. That means, mainstreaming became about flexibility, soft methods around knowledge sharing on a topic, thereby eliminating the possibility to think about gender mainstreaming in more binding, legislative terms. This kind of meaning of mainstreaming is relevant also to the case of HiAP. Mainstreaming in relation to HiAP is narrowly delineated in the way, space and scope it is supposed to be applied, and most of all, it remains a very soft, aspirational concept, unlike other mainstreamed concepts like Better Regulation.

7.3 Recycled HiAP

Both subsections above have provided some insights into potential pathways through which discursive foreground abilities can shape a malleable idea like HiAP and fit it to the prevailing EU institutional orthodoxy. Aligning HiAP with the NMG rationale—through its discursive construction as inherently about multistakeholder engagement and through its use to justify streamlining EU priorities—can confine it to a 'soft' governance space. These drifts are perhaps not surprising. Meanings are not fixed, and as such the struggle to define HiAP is a continuous one. In

[13] The word 'mainstreaming' is not invoked very often in the context of Better Regulation but is reflected in action.

turn, proponents of a more transformative HiAP have responded and are responding to these challenges by constantly reforming and redefining HiAP. In the same way as HiAP can be seen as an evolution from the Health for All idea, HiAP also evolves into new, chameleonic versions of itself. This section explores different ways in which HiAP has been 'recycled' (see Smith, 2013b, p. 81), rephrased and newly presented in response to risk of institutional co-option and watering down.

From HiAP to the Wellbeing Economy

From July to December 2019, Finland held another EU presidency. The umbrella theme for its health and social sector was the 'economy of wellbeing' (Koivisto, 2018). The Council adopted conclusions on the economy of wellbeing, which is defined as 'a policy orientation and a governance approach, which aims to put people and their well-being at the centre of policy- and decision-making' (EU Council, 2019). Furthermore, the conclusions reference HiAP and state that:

> The need to engage with cross-sectoral action is embedded in the Treaty on the Functioning of the EU and in the European Social Charter, and was referenced as part of the *Health in All Policies* approach in previous Council conclusions (2006). Pursuing the concept of Economy of Well-being *does not require new competences or structures* for EU-level actions, but it does necessitate coordinated and improved use by the Union and its Member States of their respective powers. (EU Council, 2019, p. 2, emphasis in original)

The presidency also commissioned the Organisation for Economic Co-operation and Development (OECD) to publish a conceptual framework on 'Creating opportunities for people's well-being and economic growth', which was used as a basis for the EU Council's adoption of the economy of wellbeing (All Policies for a Healthy Europe, 2019a; OECD, 2019). The framework categorises four areas to act upon to build a so-called wellbeing economy: education, healthcare, social protection and redistribution, and gender equality. Underlying the economy of wellbeing idea, is the explicit mention that GDP is not an adequate measure of countries' performance (see, e.g., Fioramonti, 2013), and that the prosperity and wellbeing of society should be evaluated based on other criteria, such as health broadly defined, and equity.

This section is interested in acknowledging the strategic shift from HiAP towards economy of wellbeing, and the shift from the word 'health' to the word 'wellbeing', as the discursive adaptation and response to some of the challenges to implement HiAP in the EU. This does not mean that what links the Wellbeing Economy agenda and HiAP together is a linear, clear-cut and coherent evolution process. An idea like the Wellbeing Economy was already existing for a long time, and one can suspect that this broad and multifaceted agenda has multiple origins. Yet within the public health circles, and in the context of EU presidencies, we are seeing a rallying behind the notion of Wellbeing Economy, as a shift from HiAP towards a new version of this old project. As put by Smith (2013b), ideas which are essentially the same can be recycled and reappear as innovative, even though they have been around for a long time. This chapter section proposes that the 'economy of wellbeing' EU presidency theme was put forward as a response to the difficulty in implementing HiAP. In the same way that 'multistakeholder HiAP' can be seen as the product of discursively modified HiAP, the 'economy of wellbeing' can be seen as a discursively modified HiAP, one that was strategically formulated to try to counter the risk of watering HiAP down. Making any predictions on whether this will or not be successful, and how 'success' should be defined in this context in the first place, is beyond the scope of this book.

Arguably, the timing of the last Finnish presidency in the second half of 2019 was not propitious to really focus on the economy of wellbeing: it occurred shortly after the election of a new EP (May 2019) and the Finnish parliamentary elections (April 2019). The new von der Leyen Commission also took office during that presidency (December 2019). And, of course, Brexit was being negotiated. This constellation of exceptional circumstances meant that the 2019 Finnish EU presidency was perhaps not as high-profile as the one in 2006. It is nevertheless interesting to reflect upon the evolution from HiAP to economy of wellbeing in terms of foreground discursive abilities, and strategies to 'recycle' and rephrase the broad aims put forward by HiAP, in a renewed way. This timeframe of change and renewal was used by a network of EU health advocacy groups to launch an initiative called 'All Policies for a Healthy Europe', which advocates for a health-focused wellbeing economy. All Policies for a Healthy Europe is multistakeholder advocacy initiative led by NGOs, not-for profit organisations, think tank, trade organisations and companies. It is funded by Johnson and Johnson, Microsoft and Randstad. This chapter does not argue that All Policies for a Healthy Europe somehow represents a radical paradigm shift. As a privately funded multi-stakeholder initiative, it is likely to present similar strucutral weaknesses as described in Chapter 5 in relation to the EU Diet Platform. An in-depth critique on the initiative is beyond the scope of this book. Instead, this advocacy initiative is drawn upon as an illustration of how the HiAP idea is continuously adapted. All Policies for a Healthy Europe explicitly builds on HiAP:

> All Policies for a Healthy Europe builds on the EU 2030 Agenda for the Sustainable Development Goals (SDGs), on the OECD's framework for Inclusive Growth, and on the work of the Finnish EU Presidency for the "Economy of Well-being" (2019) and for "Health in All Policies" (2006). (All Policies for a Healthy Europe, n.d.)

Its advocacy is based on the premise that GDP is an inadequate way to assess the performance of a country, and that goals should be directed towards fostering equity, societal wellbeing and health. It highlights the interactions between healthy people, healthy environments and 'healthy care systems', before proposing governance mechanisms that would strengthen the European Social Pillar and the inclusion of wellbeing and health across governance sectors. As such, it represents a kind of differently formulated HiAP or 'reverse HiAP', to quote one interviewee.[14] The phrasing is meant to invoke a broad vision for societal health. Substantially, it is no different from HiAP, yet it aims to close off the risk of being interpreted as 'health to be added onto each governance area', an interpretation that falls prey to both health imperialistic critiques and to a narrow conceptualisation of health.

Like HiAP, the 'economy of wellbeing' as present in the EC is a chameleonic idea, and looking at the co-option dynamics of it is beyond the scope of this book.[15] Indeed, much needs to be said about how the economy of wellbeing discourse does not challenge the economic

[14] Source: interviewee 7.

[15] An in-depth exploration of the politics of wellbeing is beyond the scope of this book. However, it is worth acknowledging that a shift from 'health' to 'wellbeing', while it makes strategic sense for the reasons argued in this chapter, does not come without its own pitfalls. Wellbeing is now often also being proposed as an indicative tool to measure countries' performance. This, of course, comes with its own challenges on how (if possible at all) to 'measure' wellbeing. The commodification of wellbeing and wellbeing as governmentality, can also be mentioned as processes worth critically reflecting upon.

paradigm of health, for example. Background documents from the 2019 Finnish EU presidency emphasise how healthier people are more innovative, productive and pay taxes (Niemi, 2019). Similarly, the OECD conceptual framework on wellbeing economy encourages the creation of public–private partnerships and stresses the important role of the private sector. As such, the economy of wellbeing as present in the EU space is not a radical idea that challenges the prevailing orthodoxy. Instead, it should be seen as a chameleonic idea too, which therefore does not fundamentally challenge prevailing orthodoxies, but which aims to act within these constraints.

From the 2006 to the 2019 Finnish presidencies, the language shifted from health to wellbeing, and there was a stronger emphasis on 'economy'. While the economy of wellbeing does not challenge the mantra that wellbeing is necessary to promote economic growth, one advantage of this kind of phrasing, one could argue, is that it targets non-health governance areas more efficiently. This very point of strategically harnessing the economic paradigm of health, but to make it work genuinely for health, was something that some Finnish interviewees[16] were far from downplaying. They did, however, caution against the risk of getting caught up in negotiations with more powerful interests, and losing sight of the health goal:

> [...] your responsibility is to bring health to the table and not just bring yourself there as an assistant for the other sectors. When you play with the more powerful people, you need to know your stuff and not forget the essence of what it is your message should put forward. (Quoted from interviewee 31)

An issue with HiAP which has been described at length in this book is its difficulty to resonate in non-health policy areas, its difficulty to reach macrosocial determinants of health. This is despite the notion that HiAP is precisely about broad definitions of health and macrosocial determinants of health. The word 'health', arguably, is a double-edged sword: on the one hand, it conjures up a kind of incontestable scientific tone, but on the other hand and for exactly these reasons, it also tends to be

For more on the politics of wellbeing, see, for example, Bache and Scott (2018), Binkley (2011) and Davies (2015).

[16] Source: interviewees 27 and 31.

boxed into a narrow scope of disease treatment and prevention, in line with the dominating pathogenic approach to public health. This is where discursively enacting a shift towards the word 'wellbeing' might be interesting, as it could offer some openings into non-health policy areas and macrosocial determinants of health. The main idea around the 'economy of wellbeing' concept is to convince that the goals and priorities of governance should be the attainment of societal wellbeing rather than economic growth.[17] The use of the word 'wellbeing', rather than health, allows for other sectors of government to feel more involved in it.[18] Similarly, it may be possible that the word 'wellbeing', because unlike 'health', it is not as strongly embedded in biomedical sciences, might lead more naturally to a political discussion around norms and values.

The economy of wellbeing idea, as suggested above, is a chameleonic idea and as such it does not challenge the economic paradigm of health. That means that, while it aims to shift priorities towards social, wellbeing goals, it does so without challenging the basic assumption that the EU needs to generate 'sustainable and inclusive' growth. Despite the structural constraints and despite the inability to fundamentally challenge ideational structures like the economic paradigm of health and even the 'multistakeholder' discourse, the economy of wellbeing idea can be seen as a continued adaptation of HiAP which seeks to respond to some of the challenges faced by HiAP. While it does not explicitly do so, it can be argued that the All Policies for a Healthy Europe initiative seeks to shape the wellbeing economy idea so as to offer solutions to some of the issues faced by HiAP (All Policies for a Healthy Europe, 2019b). Some concrete examples of these are illustrated in the Table 7.1.

Chameleonic ideas that seek to generate endogenous institutional change are fairly resilient. This does not mean that chameleonic ideas are successful[19] at changing institutions. However, proponents of chameleonic ideas like HiAP, despite their strategic discourse formulation that adopts the dominant language, are aware of the political challenges they face, such as the risk of their idea becoming co-opted and/or watered down. As a result, different discursive variations of what is essentially one same idea (Health for All, HiAP, economy of wellbeing, all propose

[17] Source: interviewees 27 and 31.

[18] Source: interviewee 32.

[19] What defines 'successful', is of course also contingent.

Table 7.1 Responses to HiAP challenges offered by the 'wellbeing economy' idea

Challenges faced by HiAP[20]	*Solutions put forward by 'wellbeing economy'*[21]
Difficulty to reach distal (political) determinants of health	– Shift from health to wellbeing – Proposal to appoint a vice-president for health – Explicit critique of GDP, the economy as a starting point
Constitutional asymmetry	– Proposal to appoint a vice-president for health – Develop a 'social imbalance procedure', in contrast to the 'macroeconomic imbalance procedure' – Include health expertise (health ministers) in the European Semester
Narrow definition of health	– Shift from health to wellbeing – Relating human, environmental and social health
Risk of watering down health on its own right	– Proposal to 'maintain a home for health within the Commission' (manifesto 1, p. 16)

a normatively identical agenda) are actively and continuously recreated, reshaped and represented so as to push for gradual institutional change, evolution 'from within'.

Wellbeing and the Degrowth Discourse

The economy of wellbeing questions the usefulness of GDP as a measure of countries' performance. That GDP is an inadequate measurement is not a radical claim, in fact even institutions like the OECD have stated it (OECD, 2019). The orthodox institutional position with respect to GDP and economic growth in the EU, does not question the absolute necessity of economic growth, but claims that it should be 'smart, inclusive and sustainable'. The full name of the overarching EUROPE

[20] Based on the analysis in this book.

[21] Based on the All Policies for a Healthy Europe manifesto.

2020 strategy (the predecessor of the European Green Deal) is 'EUROPE 2020: A strategy for smart, sustainable and inclusive growth' (European Commission, 2010). Another version of this newly packaged discourse of growth is the concept of 'green growth', which is put forward by the OECD and the World Bank as a project to 'mak[e] growth resource-efficient, cleaner and more resilient without slowing it' (World Bank, 2011, p. 2). These kinds of rebranded growth models have been criticised (Hickel & Kallis, 2020). 'Inclusive growth', for example, is a term that has been criticised for bearing little meaning. While it refers to growth that promotes employment, how exactly this 'inclusive growth' leads to poverty reduction is left unexplained (Daly, 2012). There is also a lack of clear definition of what 'green' refers to exactly in the 'green growth' concept (Rosenbaum, 2016).

In the same vein, one can also fundamentally question the 'sustainable' element of growth, and reflect on whether growth is *by definition*, unsustainable, 'green growth' representing merely capitalist green-washing (Dale, 2015). A rejection of the economic growth imperative is the basic premise behind the degrowth (or 'post-growth') idea and movement. In the current climate emergency context, where planetary boundaries are impossible to ignore, degrowth proponents challenge the idea that economies need to grow ad infinitum. Degrowth has been defined as

> [...] an equitable downscaling of production and consumption that increases human well-being and enhances ecological conditions at the local and global level in the short and in the long term. (Schneider et al., 2010, p. 511)

The degrowth idea closely relates to a normative vision in which human and environmental wellbeing are inseparable, and that the economy should work towards achieving 'harmony', rather than unlimited growth. The idea is based on the long-term view that continued growth is not sustainable and will lead (or is already leading) to a breakdown of the ecological basis of human existence. Additionally, degrowth stresses the notion that, beyond a certain threshold, economic growth no longer correlates with improved life quality and wellbeing (Easterlin et al., 2010). And finally, degrowth advocates for the need to redefine 'well-being' (Büchs & Koch, 2017). Neoclassical economic theory tends to reduce wellbeing to consumption opportunities (World Bank, 2006). A degrowth agenda would entail a need to completely rethink our wants and needs, our aspirations and how we spend our free time (i.e. develop ambitions other than accumulating wealth, and spend our free time doing things that do not involve consuming). All these deeply taken-for-granted ways of living would need to be rethought entirely, and it is not clear how such radical changes would be accepted and perceived as positive by society. Degrowth would also not be imaginable without a radical rethinking of state institutions, like the welfare system, given that currently they are engineered to function on an assumption of economic growth. Redistribution would need to be completely different for degrowth to work without jeopardising wellbeing. Degrowth is then often found alongside complementary radical ideas like universal basic income (Andersson, 2012; Kallis et al., 2012).

What is perhaps surprising to see, is that even within the EU institutional and ideational constraints, some limited and marginal spaces exist in which radical ideas like degrowth can be found. This suggests that, not only do chameleonic ideas make their way to the EU institutions, but so do—to a considerably more modest extent—some radical ideas, even though they do not resonate as loudly as chameleonic ones. Individual research papers originating from the EC's own JRC have explored and endorsed the degrowth idea. Andreoni and Galmarini (2013, 2014) have explored conceptualisations of the relationship between degrowth, social capital and wellbeing. Weiss M. and Cattaneo (2017) published a scoping review of the degrowth literature and its evolution from 2006 to 2016. The purpose of the review was to devise a degrowth research agenda, and ultimately facilitate degrowth implementation solutions. The existence of these articles is interesting in and of itself, as it shows the space for researchers in the JRC to put forward ideas that are completely outside their institutional orthodoxy.

The accent these papers put on formalising and modelling degrowth to provide concrete plans for implementation is also interesting. Weiss M. and Cattaneo (2017) highlight the evolution of the literature: they state that earlier work was mostly very philosophical, very 'social scientific', whereas 'research on degrowth has been recently branching out into more formal economics, material and energy flow accounting, and empirical case studies' (Weiss & Cattaneo, 2017, p. 222). The authors welcome this evolution, stating that '[...] the academic discourse could benefit from rigid hypotheses testing through input-output modelling, material flow analysis, life-cycle assessments, or social surveys' (p. 220). Andreoni and Galmarini (2014) provide an attempt at modelling the effects of degrowth on wellbeing. These JRC studies take a pragmatic approach to studying degrowth and do not engage as much with the philosophical debate underlying the idea. Note that is aligned with the dominance of the positivist knowledge paradigm and is yet still radical content-wise. They do very much represent an instance of discursive ability mobilised against the dominating ideational and institutional structures that take the necessity of economic growth for granted.

Another space in which the degrowth discourse is present is the EP. In September 2018, a conference on 'post-growth' was organised by ten MEPs representing five different political groups. The rationale for organising the conference was to face the problem with the growth paradigm head on and explore alternatives:

> We are surrounded by the attractive visions of 'sustainable growth', 'green growth' and promising technological solutions to environmental problems and other negative outcomes our societies produce. However, we don't dare to name the one we should blame – growth. (Post-Growth 2018 Conference, n.d.)

15 panels were organised around four key themes: the economy, the financial sector, the environment, and society. Panels included topics like basic income, tax evasion and avoidance, sustainable fiscal consolidation, to name only a few. These kinds of spaces can provide the possibility for foreground discursive articulations of dissenting ideas, even though they are located within the institutional boundaries. Arguably, the EP, given its political (in the traditional sense) nature, has more freedom to explore radical ideas than a technocratic institution like the EC. Equally, the JRC, because it is a research centre, also enjoys the same kind of relative freedom.

The point made here is not that the end of the economic growth paradigm is near. But despite the structural constraints, there are spaces for dissenting discourses, even in a rigid institution like the EU: they can take place through chameleonic ideas, which become more widely accepted and referred to, but are less radical. But there can also be smaller pockets of more radical ideas, which will likely not become part of the EC's agenda, but the existence of which still matters. Degrowth is only one example of a radical idea which can be found in rare and limited spaces in the EU, and it is one which relates to the economy of wellbeing and HiAP. Together, chameleonic ideas like HiAP and economy of wellbeing, and radical ideas like degrowth, can be seen as forming a body of agential, contesting discourses existing within the institutional boundaries and which perhaps could lead to gradual, endogenous change. Degrowth and HiAP are not the same idea. However, I want to argue here that they share common norms and values. If political, macrosocial determinants of health are taken seriously, and if neoliberalism is considered a determinant of ill-health, then degrowth and HiAP have a lot in common and can be seen as belonging to a similar type of idea in terms of content, but with differing levels of boldness. HiAP is about recognising the effects of other policy areas on health. As seen throughout the chapters, this also includes the effects of macroeconomic policies on health, in large part indirectly through their impact on inequities. Implicit in the critique of inequity-exacerbating macroeconomic system leading to ill-health is indeed the idea that a growth-centric model is both unsustainable and unfair. Instead, what HiAP stands for is a prioritisation of population health and wellbeing as more important goal, towards which the economy needs to work (rather than the other way around). Therefore, even though they are not the same ideas, HiAP and degrowth can share a common vision—depending on how HiAP is interpreted.

7.4 Conclusion: The Continuous Struggle to Define HiAP

In this final empirical chapter, we have looked at the power *over* and *through* ideas, the agential power to convince of an idea's validity, and define and attribute meaning to ideas, whether those meanings are intended to maintain institutional continuity, or whether they seek to foster endogenous institutional change. This chapter drew on the notion of chameleonic ideas to analyse the malleability of the meaning of HiAP. The first agents analysed here were the Finnish HiAP advocates who, back in 2006, shaped HiAP in a way to ensure it would become accepted in the EU space, and not be seen as too radical. Subsequently, HiAP has been reinterpreted to include multistakeholder involvement. The multistakeholder interpretation of HiAP is likely to have been promoted by industry lobbyists, too, in the same way they have been shaping the Better Regulation agenda in ways which secures them a powerful seat at the table. 'Multistakeholder HiAP' has been criticised for putting too much emphasis on involving the private sector and leading to the lifestyle drift.

Additionally, HiAP-like language is also used by the Juncker Commission to justify the need to streamline EU (economic) priorities. This tendency has led to concerns that HiAP as a slogan can be used to justify dismantling the institutional safeguards that DG SANTE represents, and instead install the equivalent of 'one health desk in every DG'. Both these instances of power *over* ideas contribute to the preservation of institutional continuity, in particular the continuity with the NMG that prevail in the EU health policy and governance area.

At the same time, HiAP is also being redefined and re-adapted. In the same way that HiAP is the continuation of the 'Health for All' agenda from the 1970s, I suggested that the theme of the 2019 Finnish EU presidency, the 'economy of wellbeing', is a continuation of the HiAP idea. The 'All Policies for a Healthy Europe' initiative advocates for an economy of wellbeing that is strong on health, and its agenda seeks solutions to challenges that HiAP has been facing in the EU. Policymakers who 'get it' can choose to advocate for a chameleonic version of this normative vision, through HiAP or the economy of wellbeing. This is another instance of power *over* ideas, where HiAP becomes constantly reshaped to address the challenges it faces.

HiAP is a very broad concept, and ultimately it is a deep-seated political vision that embraces complexity and a holistic approach to fostering wellbeing, equity and social and environmental justice. As such, it would not be coherent to consider HiAP in isolation from other, similar ideas that share broadly the same purpose, but through different avenues. The shift from HiAP to economy of wellbeing and from health to wellbeing arguably allows for more focus on the macroeconomic determinants of health through, for example, the critiques of GDP as a measurement of countries' performance. This is where the chameleonic HiAP idea connects with more radical ideas like degrowth. Even in an institutional setting like the EU, limited spaces for radical ideas like degrowth exist, albeit not in the EC per se. The extent to which degrowth and HiAP can, together, form a body of critical discourses that gradually lead to institutional change, is impossible to predict or observe without a considerable amount of hindsight.

References

All Policies for a Healthy Europe. (2019a). *The economy of well-being. Outcomes of multistakeholder roundtable*. http://healthyeurope.eu/wp-content/upl

oads/lana-downloads/2019/10/Economy-of-wellbeing_Booklet_final_Print-version.pdf. Accessed 25 March 2020.

All Policies for a Healthy Europe. (2019b). *Manifesto: Manifesto summary*. http://healthyeurope.eu/wp-content/uploads/2019/08/Healthy-Europe-Manifesto-Summary-FINAL-medium.pdf. Accessed 25 March 2020.

All Policies for a Healthy Europe. (n.d.). *'About'* [Website]. https://healthyeurope.eu/about. Accessed 25 March 2020.

Andersson, J. O. (2012, September). *Degrowth with basic income – The radical combination*. Essay written for the 14th BIEN congress, Munich. https://pdfs.semanticscholar.org/08ce/03cd105479a15cd3a9d1028564a39d822bdb.pdf. Accessed 25 March 2020.

Andreoni, V., & Galmarini, S. (2013). On the increase of social capital in degrowth economy. *Procedia—Social and Behavioral Sciences, 72*, 64–72.

Andreoni, V., & Galmarini, S. (2014). How to increase well-being in a context of degrowth. *Futures, 55*, 78–89.

Bacchi, C., & Eveline, J. (Eds.). (2010). Mainstreaming and neoliberalism: A contested relationship. In *Mainstreaming politics: Gendering practices and feminist theory* (pp. 39–60). University of Adelaide Press.

Bache, I., & Scott, K. (Eds.). (2018). *The politics of wellbeing* [eBook]. Palgrave Macmillan.

Binkley, S. (2011). Happiness, positive psychology and the program of neoliberal governmentality. *Subjectivity, 4*, 371–394.

Bruno, I., Jacquot, S., & Mandin, L. (2006). Europeanization through its instrumentation: Benchmarking, mainstreaming and the open method of co-ordination...toolbox or Pandora's box? *Journal of European Public Policy, 13*(4), 519–536.

Büchs, M., & Koch, M. (2017). *Postgrowth and wellbeing: Challenges to sustainable welfare* [eBook]. Palgrave Pivot.

Dale, G. (2015). Origins and delusions of green growth. *International Socialist Review*. Issue 97.

Daly, M. (2012). Paradigms in EU social policy: A critical account of Europe 2020. *Transfer, 18*(3), 273–284.

Davies, W. (2015). *The happiness industry: How the government and big business sold us well-being*. Verso.

Easterlin, R. A., Angelescu McVey, L., Switek, M., Sawangfa, O., & Smith Zweig, J. (2010). The happiness-income paradox revisited. *Proceedings of the National Academy of Sciences of the United States of America, 107*(52), 22463–22468.

EU Council. (2006a, 30 November and 1 December). *Council conclusions on Health in All Policies (HiAP)*. 2767th Employment, social policy, health and consumer affairs. https://ec.europa.eu/health/ph_projects/2005/action1/docs/2005_1_18_frep_a8_en.pdf. Accessed 12 November2019.

EU Council. (2006b, June 22). Council conclusions on common values and principles in European Union Health Systems. 2006/C 146/01. *Official Journal of the European Union*. https://eur-lex.europa.eu/legal-content/EN/TXT/PDF/?uri=CELEX:52006XG0622(01)&from=EN. Accessed 17 March 2020.

EU Council. (2019, October 17). *Draft council conclusions on the economy of wellbeing*. https://data.consilium.europa.eu/doc/document/ST-13171-2019-INIT/en/pdf. Accessed 25 March 2020.

European Commission. (2007a, October 23). *Together for health: A strategic approach for the EU 2008–2013* [White Paper]. Brussels. COM(2007) 630 final. https://eur-lex.europa.eu/legal-content/EN/TXT/PDF/?uri=CELEX:52007DC0630&from=EN. Accessed 12 November 2019.

European Commission. (2007b). *A strategy for Europe on nutrition, overweight and obesity related health issues* [White paper]. Brussels, 30 May. COM(2007) 279 final. https://eur-lex.europa.eu/LexUriServ/LexUriServ.do?uri=COM:2007:0279:FIN:EN:PDF. Accessed 13 November 2019.

European Commission. (2010, March 3). EUROPE 2020: A strategy for smart, sustainable and inclusive growth [Communication from the Commission] Brussels. COM(2010) 2020. https://ec.europa.eu/eu2020/pdf/COMPLET%20EN%20BARROSO%20%20%20007%20-%20Europe%202020%20-%20EN%20version.pdf. Accessed 3 April 2020.

European Commission. (2017a, October 24). *Completing the better regulation agenda* [Press Release]. PDF download available from: https://ec.europa.eu/commission/presscorner/detail/en/IP_17_4004. Accessed 12 November 2019.

European Commission. (2017b). *Better regulation 'toolbox'*. https://ec.europa.eu/info/sites/info/files/better-regulation-toolbox_2.pdf. Accessed 12 November 2019.

European Commission. (2018a). The Multiannual Financial Framework for 2021–2027: A Modern Budget for a Union that Protects, Empowers and Defends [Communication From The Commission To The European Parliament, The European Council, The Council, The European Economic And Social Committee And The Committee Of The Regions]. Brussels, 2 May. COM(2018) 321 final. https://eur-lex.europa.eu/resource.html?uri=cellar:c2bc7dbd-4fc3-11e8-be1d-01aa75ed71a1.0023.02/DOC_1&format=PDF. Accessed 12 November 2019.

European Commission. (2018b). Annex to Modern Budget for a Union that Protects, Empowers and Defends The Multiannual Financial Framework for 2021–2027 [Communication From The Commission To The European Parliament, The European Council, The Council, The European Economic And Social Committee And The Committee Of The Regions]. Brussels, 2 May COM(2018) 321 final ANNEX. https://ec.europa.eu/commis

sion/sites/beta-political/files/annex-communication-modern-budget-may 2018_en.pdf. Accessed 12 November 2019.
European Commission. (2019a). *ESI Funds for Health: Investing for a healthy and inclusive EU. Final Report.* http://www.esifundsforhealth.eu/sites/default/files/2019-03/Final%20Report%20ESI%20Funds%20for%20Health_2.pdf. Accessed 12 November 2019.
European Commission. (2019b, November 11). The European Green Deal [Communication From The Commission To The European Parliament, The European Council, The Council, The European Economic And Social Committee And The Committee Of The Regions]. Brussels. COM(2019) 640 final. https://ec.europa.eu/info/sites/info/files/european-green-deal-communication_en.pdf. Accessed 6 April 2020.
European Commission. (n.d.a). *The Recovery and Resilience Facility* [Website]. https://ec.europa.eu/info/business-economy-euro/recovery-coronavirus/recovery-and-resilience-facility_en. Accessed 3 August 2021.
Fioramonti, L. (2013). *Gross domestic problem: The politics behind the world's most powerful number.* Zed Books.
Hickel, J., & Kallis, G. (2020). Is green growth possible? *New Political Economy, 25*(4), 469–486.
Jennings, K. (2018, August 30). In Brussels, trans fats impasse nears resolution. *POLITICO.* https://www.politico.eu/article/trans-fats-limit-looms-in-brussels-targets-food-industry-health/. Accessed online 25 March 2020.
Kallis, G., Kerschner, C., & Martinez-Alier, J. (2012). The economics of degrowth. *Ecological Economics, 84*, 172–180.
Kemm, J. (2001). Health impact assessment: A tool for healthy public policy. *Health Promotion International, 16*(1), 79–85.
Koivisto, T. (2018, November 23). *The Finnish EU Presidency* [PowerPoint Presentation]. Finnish Ministry of Social Affairs and Health. https://ec.europa.eu/health/sites/health/files/non_communicable_diseases/docs/ev_20181106_co02_en.pdf. Accessed 25 March 2020.
Koivusalo, M. (2010). The state of Health in All Policies (HiAP) in the European Union: Potential and pitfalls. *Journal of Epidemiology and Community Health, 64*(6), 500–503.
Koivusalo, M. (2019, April 14). HiAP [PowerPoint presentation]. Brown bag lunch presentation series, Social and Health Policy Group at the University of Tampere, Finland.
Lynch, J. (2020). *Regimes of inequality—The political economy of health and wealth.* Cambridge University Press.
Mykhalovskiy, E., Frohlich, K. L., Poland, B., Di Ruggiero, E., Rock, M. J., & Comer, L. (2019). Critical social science with public health: Agonism, critique and engagement. *Critical Public Health, 29*(5), 522–533.

Niemi, V. (2019). *Economy of wellbeing in the EU: People's wellbeing fosters economic growth.* Background Document. https://eu2019.fi/en/backgrounders/economy-of-wellbeing. Accessed 25 March 2020.

OECD. (2019, June 21). *The economy of well-being: Executive Summary of the OECD Background paper on "Creating opportunities for people's well-being and economic growth"*. https://data.consilium.europa.eu/doc/document/ST-10414-2019-INIT/en/pdf. Accessed 25 March 2020.

Ollila, E., Ståhl, T., Wismar, M., Lahtinen, E., Melkas, T., Melkas, T., & Leppo, K. (2006). *Health in All Policies in the European Union and its member states* [Policy Brief]. https://ec.europa.eu/health/ph_projects/2005/action1/docs/2005_1_18_frep_a4_en.pdf. Accessed 11 November 2019.

Rosenbaum, E. (2016). Some observations on green growth. *JRC Science for Policy Report*. https://publications.jrc.ec.europa.eu/repository/bitstream/JRC103728/lbna28228enn.pdf. Accessed 25 March 2020.

Schneider, F., Kallis, G., & Martinez-Alier, J. (2010). Crisis or opportunity? Economic degrowth for social equity and ecological sustainability. Introduction to this special issue. *Journal of Cleaner Production, 18*(6), 511–518.

Smith, K. E. (2010). Research, policy and funding—Academic treadmills and the squeeze on intellectual space. *The British Journal of Sociology, 61*(1), 176–195.

Smith, K. E. (2012). Fools, facilitators and Flexians: Academic identities in marketised environments. *Higher Education Quarterly, 66*(2), 155–173.

Smith, K. E. (2013a). *Beyond evidence-based policy in public health: The interplay of ideas*. Palgrave Macmillan.

Smith, K. E. (2013b). Institutional filters: The translation and re-circulation of ideas about health inequalities within policy. *Policy & Politics, 41*(1), 81–100.

Smith, K. E. (2014). The politics of ideas: The complex interplay of health inequalities research and policy. *Science and Public Policy, 41*(5), 561–574.

Smith, K. E., & Joyce, K. E. (2012). Capturing complex realities: Understanding efforts to achieve evidence-based policy and practice in public health. *Evidence & Policy, 8*(1), 57–78.

Smith, K. E., Fooks, G., Gilmore, A. B., Collin, J., & Weishaar, H. (2015). Corporate coalitions and policymaking in the European Union: How and why British American Tobacco promoted 'Better Regulation.' *Journal of Health Politics, Policy and Law, 40*(2), 325–372.

Ståhl, T., Wismar, M., Ollila, E., Lahtinen, E., & Leppo, K., (Eds.). (2006). *Health in all policies: Prospects and potentials*. Ministry of Social Affairs and Health, Finland.

Synnevåg, E. S., Amdam, R., & Fosse, E. (2018). Public health terminology: Hindrance to a Health in All Policies approach? *Scandinavian Journal of Public Health, 46*(1), 68–73.

Tselengidis, A., & Östergren, P. (2019). Lobbying against sugar taxation in the European Union: Analysing the lobbying arguments and tactics of stakeholders in the food and drink industries. *Scandinavian Journal of Public Health, 47*, 565–575.

WebsitePost-Growth 2018 Conference. (n.d.). *Why post-growth?* https://www.postgrowth2018.eu/why/. Accessed 25 March 2020.

Weiss, C. H. (1977). Research for policy's sake: The enlightenment function of social research. *Policy Analysis, 3*(4), 531–545.

Weiss, C. H. (1979). The many meanings of research utilization. *Public Administration Review, 39*(5), 426–431.

Weiss, M., & Cattaneo, C. (2017). Degrowth—Taking stock and reviewing an emerging academic paradigm. *Ecological Economics, 137*, 220–230.

World Bank. (2006). *Where is the wealth of nations? Measuring capital for the 21st century*. http://documents.worldbank.org/curated/en/287171468323724180/pdf/348550REVISED0101Official0use0ONLY1.pdf

World Bank. (2011). *From growth to green growth a framework*. http://documents.worldbank.org/curated/en/264561468163484844/pdf/WPS5872.pdf. Accessed 25 March 2020.

CHAPTER 8

Conclusion

HiAP has little *intrinsic* meaning. Its interpretation is a continuous political, normative struggle, shaped by intentional discursive strategies, prevailing institutional structures and more fluid, cognitive systems of meanings. We've seen in this book how the asymmetries in EU institutional structures render a HiAP uptake, as imagined by Finnish HiAP advocates, difficult. But beyond constitutional asymmetry, barriers to institutional change are also ingrained in commonly accepted ways to conceptualise certain issues, like health, NCDs or even what constitutes usable scientific evidence. This suggests a more pervasive, yet less monolithically neoliberal EU. With the growing understanding of macrosocial determinants of health, and their political nature, the relevance of the EU activities to public health is becoming more visible. At the same time, public health is yet again confronted with tensions related to its embeddedness in a positivist approach to scientific evidence as neutral and its recognition that health promotion is political. This raises challenges for how the research/policy relationship is to be understood. HiAP is an attempt to work around those tensions, without addressing them explicitly. Whether the ongoing recycling of HiAP can be deemed successful remains debatable and depends on the extent of the change one was expecting.

C. Godziewski, *The Politics of Health Promotion*, Palgrave Studies in Science, Knowledge and Policy, https://doi.org/10.1007/978-3-030-97870-9_8

8.1 Health Promotion Is Political

One recurring theme in this book has been the accent on the political and normative nature of health promotion. What I mean by 'political' is not synonymous with party politics. Rather, political here is used to describe something which produces power dynamics that structure social relations. Rather than looking at technical implementation of health impact assessments or other approaches to considering health in other policies, we explored the institutional, ideational and discursive power dynamics that shape the meaning(s) of health promotion in the EU and in turn, the scope of HiAP. The arguments developed in this book are also inherently and inevitably value-driven, driven by a concern for fostering a healthier, more just and sustainable EU in which population emancipation and well-being is a goal in itself (rather than a means to another goal). The starting point has been to consider seriously the research on neoliberalism, ill-health, and health inequity and engage with the implications in terms of health promotion: if neoliberalism is considered a determinant of ill-health and health inequity, then health promotion needs to be radically redefined to encompass more explicitly normative commitments to health, as well as social and environmental equity. Doing this would broaden the scope of what is understood as constituting health promotion. And it would broaden the scope of HiAP and the areas HiAP has relevance to.

Yet 'broad and normative' is not how HiAP (or health promotion, for that matter) is generally understood. Why not? This is a central puzzle of this book. I suggest that the answers pertain to some extent to how EU institutions are structured asymmetrically and are ideationally sustained. For HiAP to be understood in a more 'social' way, the EU would need to be more social in its governance structures and rationality. But at the same time, we also need to seek answers to this puzzle in the public health discipline itself. Despite the vast amount of research on macrosocial determinants of health, including the growing literature on the so-called commercial determinants of health, I suggest that there remains a lack of meaningful engagement by much (though of course not all) of the public health field with questions of political economy and theorisation of power. I argue that this relates to epistemological tensions in that field, between the desire of parts of public health research to seek authority and influence by attempting to place its evidence 'above politics' on the one hand. Yet on the other hand, there is a recognition that the determinants of today's biggest public health burdens are inherently political, and that offering evidence is not enough to catalyse change.

This book explored how these tensions play out in the context of the EU and the HiAP agenda. The EU is a particularly interesting governance space to look at, given its (the European Commission's in particular) propensity to a technocratic, depoliticised approach to governing markets more than social matters. Yet the confluence and intimate relation between what is commonly considered apolitical and what is commonly considered political are becoming impossible to ignore. The very distinction between 'political' versus 'apolitical' is a product of power. Consequently, one overarching argument made in this book is a call for more engagement with the ontological diversity in public health scholarship. Critical social scientific approaches in public health offer a sophisticated picture of the interconnectedness of public health determinants, and how power operates in relation to them. Taking seriously the normative nature of macrosocial determinants of health makes visible the need to study health (including health promotion and HiAP) from a critical social scientific perspective.

Taking a broad, normative conceptualisation of health promotion and viewing neoliberalism as a determinant of health also makes the relevance of EU (non-health) competencies to health become more visible. Therefore, another overarching argument in this book is that health should feature more prominently in EU studies, not only because of spill over effects, but also because of the spaces in which macrosocial determinants of health are shaped. A possible reason EU health promotion is an under-represented area of study relates to the way in which health promotion is normally defined in a restrictive way, given its official status as primarily a member state competence. But what is 'health promotion'? When considering the complexity turn in NCD prevention and health promotion, the relevance of HiAP at EU level and the relevance of EU public health promotion as a research object make much more sense: competencies related to Single Market integration through to economic governance *are* macrosocial determinants of health. This raises the question of how indirect health impacts of EU non-health competencies can be made more visible, discussed and acted upon, and even whether we should talk about 'health' or 'wellbeing'.

It is also useful to emphasise the need for more research on EU health, because EU studies do not neutrally observe the EU as an entity existing in a vacuum. Rather, EU studies, how the EU is theorised, talked about, researched and criticised, shape the EU as a social construction. Challenging orthodox conceptualisations of what the EU is and what it does (Ryner, 2012), exposing the subtle, overlooked power dynamics and political effects from a critical perspective, is in itself political—and necessary for promoting institutional change. Studying EU health promotion therefore also has relevance to the broader debate on economic versus social Europe. The critical approach to EU studies adopted here points to the need to look beyond constitutional asymmetry when investigating the failures to promote a more social Europe. It also draws attention to the need to look beyond the soft/hard governance asymmetries and conventional institutional factors.

8.2 HiAP in the EU: Structural Barriers and Malleable Ideas

HiAP, ultimately, has little intrinsic meaning. Its introduction to the EU does not automatically lead to a clearly defined, undeniable and immediate change. The EU presents considerable institutional and ideational obstacles to HiAP, and these are political obstacles more than technical ones. As they stand, the asymmetrical EU institutional structures are unlikely to enable the kind of HiAP that many of its advocates are hoping for. Governance areas that are perceived as being relevant to HiAP tend to be situated in the realm of soft governance and pertain mostly to 'proximal' determinants of health often associated with the behavioural paradigm of health. This is visible, for example, in the EU Diet Platform and the HLG. On the other hand, those governance areas that impact macrosocial determinants of health (such as social inequity or the food system) are perceived to be less relevant to HiAP and are dealt with through harder means of governance. This was visible through the very limited policy space for health in Single Market regulations, in the CAP, and in EU economic governance. Finally, the EU meta-regulatory landscape also reflects constitutional asymmetrical biases, as illustrated through the example of the Better Regulation agenda and DG SANTE's Strategic Plan for 2016–2020.

This asymmetry does manifest not only through institutional structures in a conventional sense, but also cognitively, through established systems of meanings, so-called background ideational structures. The power and authority that certain ideas have, their 'taken-for-granted' character and their exclusionary power towards dissenting ideas also represent a challenge to HiAP-minded institutional change. Exploring these factors requires a more constructivist, discursive analytical approach, such as looking at the normative underpinning of paradigms informing problem frames. We have seen how—notwithstanding the link between demographic change and NCD prevalence—framing NCDs as a problem of 'ageing of populations' obscures the social and inequality dimensions of NCDs by portraying them as the inevitable result of increased life expectancy, i.e. of progress. On the one hand, the NCDs 'crisis' is presented as a matter of threat posed by 'a tsunami of elderly people' that may lead to the collapse of member states health and pension systems. This can then serve to justify austerity measures and budget cuts, as well as pressures to come up with individual self-management solutions. On the other hand, the ageing population framing also mobilises solutions centred around personalised medicine, eHealth, mHealth and biomedical innovation: health as a profitable market. The way in which 'evidence' is framed, and the requirement for it to be SMART is also problematic when dealing with a concept like HiAP, which cannot necessarily be measured and which is inherently normative. Again, this point is quite tricky because of the epistemological tensions in public health, and the tensions between the authority of 'normative neutrality' and the political nature of health promotion—the risk of being dismissed if one's ideas appear 'too normative'. This tension is at the core of the research/policy relationship and manifests beyond the case of health mainstreaming.

For HiAP to have a chance at bringing about any sort of gradual and slow change, it would need to be continuously renegotiated and recycled. This would require continuous engagement with its meaning and definition, as a power struggle, to avoid its watering down or its 'co-option'. This risk was illustrated in how HiAP became actively redefined in the EU space, so as to fit the NMG agenda: on the one hand, through the ambiguity of the term 'sector', the EU interpreted HiAP as inherently about engaging all stakeholders, an interpretation vehemently contested by the Finnish HiAP advocates interviewed. At the same time, there was a worry among some interviewees that HiAP language was being used to justify dismantling the institutional safeguards for health and further streamlining EC economic priorities. This relates to the ambiguity of the term 'mainstreaming', and how it refers to a technocratic NMG tool in the case, for example, of gender mainstreaming, whereas it refers to something much more all-encompassing and deep seated in the case of, say, Better Regulation.

At the same time, the 'economy of wellbeing' agenda of the 2019 Finnish EU presidency can be seen as a continuation of the HiAP agenda, seeking to address some of the challenges faced since 2006. The shift from using the term 'health' to using the term 'wellbeing'—while not without its own challenges—can perhaps allow other governance areas to be more invested in taking it up, as wellbeing is a broader goal to which more governance areas will perceive they have relevance. Similarly, by being less directly associated with the biomedical realm, 'wellbeing' may allow for a more explicit discussion around politics, norms and values. Finally, the 'economy of wellbeing' phrasing *could* also lead to a discussion of the inadequacy of the current macroeconomic model, for example critiquing the GDP measurement. The economy of wellbeing, like HiAP, is a chameleonic idea and therefore does not fundamentally or radically challenge the institutional orthodoxy. But other, more radical versions of broadly this idea exist, such as the degrowth movement. Even within a conventional and rigid institution like the EU, spaces for the degrowth idea do exist, notably in the JRC and the EP. While degrowth is unlikely to become widely accepted in the EU (at least in the foreseeable future), the presence of radical, marginal ideas, together with chameleonic—more widespread but much less radical—ideas is useful to highlight to remain aware that the EU is not *monolithically* neoliberal. The extent to which those ideas can bring about meaningful change, however, is difficult to determine.

8.3 Future Research Agenda

We are in the middle of the Von der Leyen European Commission presidency, the beginning of which happened to coincide with a major health crisis. It is fair to say that the EU governance landscape, including in health, is likely to experience considerable changes. On the one hand, we should keep a close eye on the unfolding of the European Green Deal (European Commission, 2019a) agenda and the extent to which it successfully socialises and 'environmentalises' EU economic governance tools and other EU competencies. Arguably, the European Green Deal, while it is at an early stage, and without suggesting that it embodies a radical paradigm shift, does look like progress compared to the Juncker priorities. This gradual slow change may be attributable to, on the one hand, the agency of the individuals making up the new commission, and on the other hand, the presence of discourses (within and outside the EU institutions) that push for the prioritisation of wellbeing, social justice and environmental sustainability. There seems to be, at least at first sight, a stronger focus on aligning EU action with the sustainable development goals, and while it does not challenge the economic growth paradigm, it aims to decouple economic growth from resource use (European Commission, 2019a, p.2). It also states 'put[*ting*] sustainability and the well-being of citizens at the centre of economic policy' as a goal (p. 3). The European Green Deal also contains concrete policy examples, timelines, an investment plan and dedicated funds to work towards these goals (European Commission, 2019a, 2019b, 2020a, 2020b). It will be interesting to see whether shifts from HiAP towards wellbeing economy, and the European Green Deal's role in streamlining these priorities, might affect DGs other than SANTE, if at all. In the EC, HiAP is perceived as mostly relevant to DG SANTE. This is paradoxical, because HiAP is precisely about the health impact of non-health policies. How will non-health DGs be affected if wellbeing promotion becomes a priority to be streamlines across DGs? Without being unrealistically optimistic, one can reflect on the extent to which the establishment of the European Green Deal represents an outcome of slow, endogenous institutional change, and whether the discursive weight of chameleonic ideas like HiAP and the economy of wellbeing has contributed to this slow change.

But what happens to more radical ideas, and how do they achieve change? Here, I suggest more research around the salience of the 'degrowth' (or post-growth) concept in connection to public health and wellbeing would be needed. While we have looked at the resonance of HiAP as an idea at EU level, we have yet to delve into exploring what the EU could look like, concretely, if HiAP was meaningfully implemented as a normative project rather than as a technical instrument. In order to develop this kind of research agenda, it is fundamental to work towards redefining what counts as 'health promotion'. Exploring the connection between such radically broad conceptualisations of health promotion as put forward here, and the idea of degrowth (or post-growth) makes a lot of sense, because of the ultimately normative convergence between trying to improve macrosocial determinants of health and degrowth considerations. Radical ideas like degrowth that challenge the dominant macroeconomic model are driven by what is ultimately the same vision for a more just, and equitable world, one that strives for a meaningful purpose beyond consumption, capital accumulation and economic growth. However, the intersection between public health and degrowth has yet to be researched more in detail (see, for example, the work of Büchs & Koch, 2017): how to ensure the theoretical link between degrowth and wellbeing actually holds in practice. This is far from obvious, given that current structures like welfare states in Western countries are built on the premise of economic growth. At the same time, cultural and social perceptions of what represents wellbeing, aspirations, goals and beliefs regarding how to achieve wellbeing are also deeply embedded in a capitalist worldview.

Finally, it is worth reflecting more broadly on the impact that the current pandemic might have on the importance given to health on political agenda, but also and importantly, *how* this renewed attention on health might take place. Will we be able to witness some broader changes in political rationality towards more global, intersectional social justice, wealth redistribution and equity? Or will the changes be driven more by protectionism and border securitisation? In the context of COVID-19, some have called for 'more Europe', arguing that coordinated and unified responses to cross-border health threats at a union level would be more efficient than atomised state-level responses (Costa-Font, 2020; Renda & Castro, 2020). Better collaboration on data gathering, surveillance of cross-border health threats and pandemic preparedness are important and clearly necessary. This seems to be one of the key priorities of the EU's 'European Health Union' project which features, as a central element, the establishment of the EU Health Emergency preparedness and Response Authority (HERA) (European Commission, 2021).

However, what this book has aimed to draw attention to is that political economy, climate change, the global food system, NCDs and the increased likelihood of pandemics are all related issues that need to be viewed holistically and normatively (Rushton, 2019). Will the current pandemic lead to a focus onto the broad political economic root causes of public illness, the macrosocial determinants of health? Will it make it impossible to ignore the connections between neoliberal capitalism and health? Despite NCDs and infectious pandemics being two very different public health problems, they are not unrelated in terms of one of their main underlying political determinants: inequity and precarity. At a time when individual responsibility narratives in relation to 'healthy lifestyle promotion' are under ever-growing criticism, when solutions to the destructive consequences of political decisions continue to be pushed into the realm of individual action, the COVID-19 pandemic is blatantly exposing the limits of disembedded free market economies and underscoring the importance of strong social and environmental protection. Trying to make sure these relationships do not go unnoticed, trying to make sure they become politicised and contested, is both an implication of this book and a long-term future research agenda. Before thinking about *more* Europe, we need to think about a *different*, more socially progressive and healthy Europe.

References

Büchs, M., & Koch, M. (2017). *Postgrowth and wellbeing: Challenges to sustainable welfare* [eBook]. Palgrave Pivot.

Costa-Font, J. (2020, March 24). *Europe's failure to address Covid-19 shows the need for a European 'health citizenship'*. LSE EUROPP Blog. https://blogs.lse.ac.uk/europpblog/2020/03/24/europes-failure-to-address-covid-19-shows-the-need-for-a-european-health-citizenship/. Accessed 22 September 2021.

European Commission. (2019a, November 11). The European Green Deal [Communication From The Commission To The European Parliament, The European Council, The Council, The European Economic And Social Committee And The Committee Of The Regions]. Brussels, 11 November 2019 . COM(2019) 640 final. https://ec.europa.eu/info/sites/info/files/european-green-deal-communication_en.pdf. Accessed 6 April 2020.

European Commission. (2019b, November 11). Annex to the European Green Deal [Communication From The Commission To The European Parliament, The European Council, The Council, The European Economic And Social Committee and The Committee of The Regions]. Brussels. COM(2019) 640 final. https://ec.europa.eu/info/sites/info/files/european-green-deal-communication-annex-roadmap_en.pdf. Accessed 6 April 2020.

European Commission. (2020a, January 14). Sustainable Europe Investment Plan European Green Deal Investment Plan [Communication From The Commission To The European Parliament, The Council, The European Economic And Social Committee And The Committee Of The Regions]. Brussels. COM(2020) 21 final. https://eur-lex.europa.eu/legal-content/EN/TXT/PDF/?uri=CELEX:52020DC0021&from=EN. Accessed 6 April 2020.

European Commission. (2020b, January 14). Proposal for a Regulation of the European Parliament and of The Council establishing the Just Transition Fund. Brussels. COM(2020) 22 final. https://eur-lex.europa.eu/resource.html?uri=cellar:b82780d8-3771-11ea-ba6e-01aa75ed71a1.0003.02/DOC_1&format=PDF. Accessed 6 April 2020.

European Commission. (2021). Introducing HERA, the European Health Emergency preparedness and Response Authority, the next step towards completing the European Health Union. COM(2021) 576 final. https://ec.europa.eu/health/system/files/2021-09/hera_2021_comm_en_0.pdf (europa.eu). Accessed 10 January 2022.

Renda, A., & Castro, R. (2020). Towards stronger EU governance of health threats after the COVID-19 pandemic. *European Journal of Risk Regulation, 11*(2), 273–282.

Rushton, S. (2019). *Security and public health: Pandemics and politics in the contemporary world*. Polity Press.

Ryner, M. (2012). Financial crisis, orthodoxy and heterodoxy in the production of knowledge about the EU. *Millennium., 40*(3), 647–673.

List of Interviewees

Interviewee number	*Interviewee type*	*Date*	*Location*
1	EU NGO representative	08/03/2018	Brussels
2	Representative for an EU food and drink industry	09/03/2018	Brussels
3	EC official	22/03/2018; 04/06/2018	Luxembourg, Luxembourg
4	Industry representative	26/03/2018	Brussels
5	NGO representative	26/03/2018	Via Skype
6	Industry representative	27/03/2018	Brussels
7	EC official	06/04/2018	Luxembourg
8	EC official	06/04/2018	Luxembourg
9	EU NGO representative	10/04/2018	Brussels
10	Industry representative	13/04/2018	Brussels
11	EC official	16/04/2018	By telephone
12	EU NGO representative	05/04/2018	Brussels
13	EU NGO representative	01/06/2018	Brussels
14	EU NGO representative	04/04/2018	Brussels
15	Member state health ministry representative	12/04/2018	Email exchange
16	Former EC official	17/04/2018	Brussels
17	Member state health ministry representative	18/04/2018	By telephone

(continued)

C. Godziewski, *The Politics of Health Promotion*, Palgrave Studies in Science, Knowledge and Policy, https://doi.org/10.1007/978-3-030-97870-9

(continued)

Interviewee number	*Interviewee type*	*Date*	*Location*
18	Member state health ministry representative	19/04/2018	Luxembourg
19	Member state health ministry representative	19/04/2018	Luxembourg
20	EU health advocate	20/04/2018	Luxembourg
21	Member of the European Parliament assistant	28/05/2018	Brussels
22	EC official	04/06/2018	Luxembourg
23	Research and evaluation company representative	11/06/2018	Brussels
24	Member of the European Parliament	19/06/2018	Brussels
25	Former MEP assistant	22/06/2018	Luxembourg
27	Member state health ministry representative	04/07/2018; 23/04/2019	Via Skype; Helsinki
28	EC official	09/07/2018	By telephone
29	EC official	09/07/2018	By telephone
30	Finnish NGO representative	18/04/2019	Helsinki
31	Member state health ministry representative	23/04/2019	Helsinki
32	Finnish public health researcher	29/04/2019	Tampere
33	Finnish health policymaker	17/04/2019	Helsinki
34	Finnish health policymaker	17/04/2019	Helsinki
35	Finnish health policymaker	17/04/2019	Helsinki

Index

C. Godziewski, *The Politics of Health Promotion*, Palgrave Studies in Science, Knowledge and Policy, https://doi.org/10.1007/978-3-030-97870-9

FSC
www.fsc.org
MIX
Papier | Fördert
gute Waldnutzung
FSC® C083411

Kolibri 360 GmbH
Ferdinand-Jühlke-Straße 7
99095 Erfurt, Deutschland
produktsicherheit@kolibri360.de